Anatomy Vivas for the Intercollegiate MRCS

Anatomy Vivas for the Intercollegiate MRCS

Nick A. Aresti

Core Surgical Trainee in the London Deanery, London, UK

Manoj Ramachandran

Consultant Orthopaedic and Trauma Surgeon (Paediatric and Young Adult), Barts Health NHS Trust, London, England and Honorary Senior Lecturer, William Harvey Research Institute, Barts and The London School of Medicine and Dentistry, Queen Mary's, University of London, UK

Mark D. Stringer

Professor of Anatomy at the University of Otago, Dunedin, New Zealand and Chair of the Anatomy Committee, Royal Australasian College of Surgeons

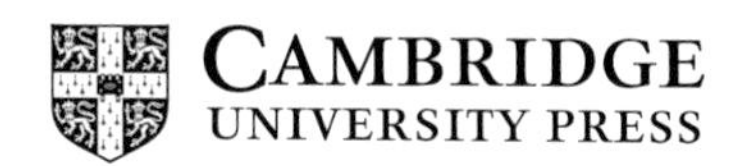

CAMBRIDGE UNIVERSITY PRESS
Cambridge, New York, Melbourne, Madrid, Cape Town,
Singapore, São Paulo, Delhi, Mexico City

Cambridge University Press
The Edinburgh Building, Cambridge CB2 8RU, UK

Published in the United States of America by Cambridge University Press, New York

www.cambridge.org
Information on this title: www.cambridge.org/9781107672994

First published 2012

Printed and bound in the United Kingdom by the MPG Books Group

A catalogue record for this publication is available from the British Library

Library of Congress Cataloging-in-Publication Data
Anatomy vivas for the intercollegiate MRCS / [edited by] Nick Aresti, Manoj Ramachandran,
Mark Stringer.
p. cm.
ISBN 978-1-107-67299-4 (Paperback)
1. Human anatomy–Examinations, questions, etc. 2. Anatomy, Surgical and topographical–Examinations, questions, etc. I. Aresti, Nick. II. Ramachandran, Manoj. III. Stringer, Mark.
QM32.A658 2012
612.0076–dc23

2012008942

ISBN 978-1-107-67299-4 Paperback

Dedicated to my parents, Ari and Niki
Nick Aresti

For my beautiful girls Joanna, Izzy and Mia
Manoj Ramachandran

To my wonderful children Paul, Stephen and Catherine
Mark Stringer

Contents

Authors

Nick A. Aresti **BSc MBBS MRCS FHEA**
Core Surgical Trainee, London Deanery, London

Manoj Ramachandran **BSc(Hons) MBBS(Hons) MRCS(Eng) FRCS(Tr&Orth)**
Consultant Orthopaedic and Trauma Surgeon (Paediatric and Young Adult), Barts Health NHS Trust, London, England and Honorary Senior Lecturer, William Harvey Research Institute, Barts and The London School of Medicine and Dentistry, Queen Mary's, University of London, London

Mark D. Stringer **BSc MS FRCP FRCS FRCSPaed FRCSEd**
Professor of Anatomy at the Department of Anatomy, University of Otago, Dunedin, New Zealand, Chairman of the Anatomy Committee, Royal Australasian College of Surgeons

Acknowledgments

We would like to thank several people for their contribution to this book.

- Nick Dunton, Senior Commissioning Editor and Rob Sykes, Assistant Editor, Cambridge University Press.

  Nick and Rob were ever present, providing expert opinion and advice. Without their help and enthusiasm, this book would not have been possible.
- Dr Catherine Molyneux, Director of Anatomical Studies, Queen Mary's School of Medicine and Dentistry.

  Cathy not only provided many of the fantastic images seen in this book, but also granted us access to the anatomy laboratory at Queen Mary's University to take photographs.
- Brynley Crosado (Prosector) and Chris Smith (Curator) of the W. D. Trotter Anatomy Museum at the University of Otago, for the inclusion of selected images.
- Stephanie Constantine.

  We would like to thank Stephanie for her help, support and modelling.
- Panos Michaelides.

  Panos provided his expertise and support during preparation of the images.
- Bhavin Upadhyay.

  Bhavin provided us with some of the radiographic images seen in this book.

Introduction

The MRCS (Membership of the Royal College of Surgeons) exam has undergone drastic changes in recent years, one of the most significant being the way in which anatomy is examined. As a candidate sitting the exam it is essential that you spend the necessary time learning your anatomy in sufficient detail not only to pass the exam, but also to continue your surgical training. In the process it is vital that you understand the exam structure and adapt your learning style accordingly.

Although this book has been designed primarily as a revision guide and a learning tool, it has been put together in a manner that is very similar to the structure of the anatomy vivas in the exam. The questions are clinically orientated and are based around themes and clinical scenarios. Photographs of cadavers and prosections, simple diagrams, radiography and photographs of actors are all incorporated into the text to ensure the questions are as similar as possible to the questions in the actual exam.

Most of the topics which have been examined in the new exam system are covered in significant detail in this book. It is no secret that the College is only able to write so many questions and so there is a lot of repetition. Learning the contents of this book will therefore aid your performance in the exam. You must however be wary that you may well be the subject of a completely new anatomy viva station, so do not get lulled into a false sense of security and only learn the topics that have come up in the past.

Use this book in combination with anatomy textbooks and video tutorials. You may never have been examined in the format employed in the exam, particularly on basic science topics. In preparation therefore, practice reciting your answers out loud to colleagues, friends, family or even pets if you have to.

No doubt you will have many a sleepless night and anxious moments in the lead up to your exam. As someone who has recently been through the exam and then helped friends through, let this reassure you: as long as you study hard and take heed of the advice presented here and elsewhere, you stand a good chance of passing. The new exam is a fair test of those who are properly prepared.

The MRCS exam

To become a member of the Royal College of Surgeons, you must pass part A and part B of the exam (and of course part with the subscription and annual fees). Part A involves two multiple-choice papers, and part B is an Objective Structured Clinical Examination (OSCE) consisting of 18 examined stations alongside preparation and rest stations. All stations are now 'manned', i.e. have an examiner present who will be asking you questions. Note that the new-style system did originally have some 'unmanned' stations before the exam was slightly revamped.

Each OSCE station will examine you on one or more of four broad content areas. You receive a mark for each area and must pass all of them in order to receive an overall pass. The four areas are:

- *Anatomy and surgical pathology*
- *Applied surgical science and critical care*
- *Communication skills in giving and receiving information and history taking*
- *Clinical and procedural skills.*

When applying for the exam, you will be asked to pick specialty context areas which will influence the content of part of your exam. This is designed to meet the emerging intention of trainees with regard to their chosen subspecialty. The four areas as stipulated by the examinations board are:

- *Head and neck*
- *Trunk and thorax*
- *Limbs (including spine)*
- *Neuroscience.*

It should be noted that the specialty area named 'trunk and thorax' is a misnomer: the term 'trunk' of course includes the thorax.

You will be asked to pick a first, second and third choice specialty. Your first choice will be examined in three stations: an anatomy/pathology viva station, a history taking station and a physical examination station. Your second specialty choice will be examined in two stations: a history taking station and a physical examination station. Finally your third specialty choice will be examined only in a physical examination station.

The anatomy and surgical pathology broad content area is normally examined in 4 of the 18 stations. They are typically the same style in every exam and are laid out as follows:

1. *An anatomy viva based on the first-choice specialty area.*
   This, the only specialty-specific station in the anatomy and pathology broad content area, is a complicated anatomy viva which is in more detail than the generic anatomy stations.
2. *Two 'generic' anatomy viva stations.*
   The theme of the generic stations is not related to the specialty choices you pick, and may therefore be based on any of the four specialty choices. Therefore if you pick limbs, thorax and neurosciences for your specialty choices, you may still get a viva based on the larynx or thyroid gland (i.e. head

and neck). So far, we know of no-one who has been examined on neuroanatomy in a generic anatomy station after *not* picking neurosciences as their first choice specialty.

3. *A pathology viva station.*
   All pathology stations involve a structured viva independent of the specialty choices.

What does this mean for the exam and for your revision? As already touched on, it is a common misconception that you only need to learn the anatomy relevant to your specialty choices. Other than detailed neuroanatomy, all anatomy must be learnt in sufficient detail. We do however recommend that you ensure the anatomy relating to your first-choice specialty is your strongest topic, as you are guaranteed a grilling in this area!

Anatomy is only examined in 3 of the 18 stations. Other areas such as communication skills carry approximately the same weight in the exam. It would be wise to split your revision time between your educational needs with the structure of the exam in mind.

With regard to the rest of the exam, a few words of advice: pathologies presented are not the rare and unusual conditions suggested by other commonly used MRCS revision guides. They are diseases which you will almost certainly have come across in your clinical practice. For example, osteoarthritic knees, or lower limbs with peripheral vascular disease are very common in the limbs and spine stations; thyroid nodules and salivary gland swellings are common in the head and neck stations; and incisional hernias and 'acute' abdomens in the trunk stations.

Another commonly failed broad content area is the critical care section. The contents of this area is beyond the remit of the book. However we can say that the questioning follows the logical sequences which can be found in the CCrISP (Care of the Critically Ill Surgical Patient) course-books.

In summary, learn your anatomy, learn it well and practise describing what you have learnt. Understand and appreciate the structure of the exam and modify your revision accordingly. Do not ignore any of the possible topics that may come up in your exam, be it anatomy of the parotid gland or the seven hand-washing steps. Finally, be confident in your knowledge and confident in your answers.

The very best of luck!

1

Limbs and vertebral column questions

Question 1

Scenario:
A young man is walking along a road when a car travelling at 30 mph (48 km/h) drives past. The side-view mirror strikes his right shoulder and he sustains an injury to his humerus.

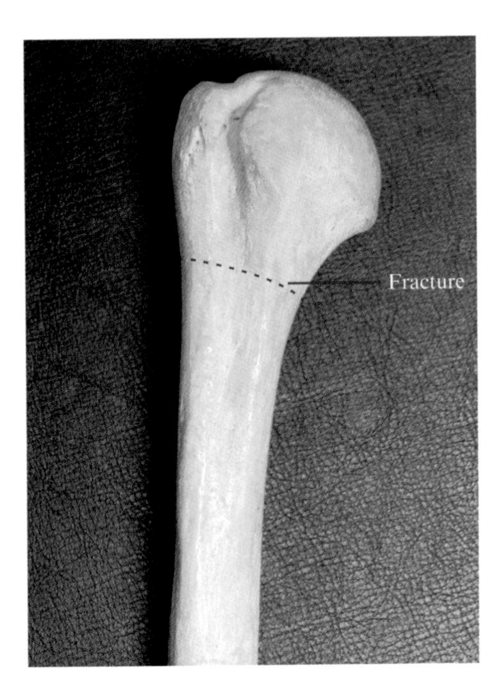

Image 1.1

With regards to Image 1.1:

I. Identify the greater tubercle.
II. Identify the lesser tubercle.
III. Identify the anatomical neck of the humerus.
IV. Identify the surgical neck of the humerus.

A radiograph shows a fracture at the site marked on Image 1.1.

V. What nerve is at risk following this type of injury?
VI. What clinical features would be present if the nerve was damaged?
VII. Which nerve runs in the spiral groove of the humerus?
VIII. If a fracture was to injure this nerve, what clinical findings might be expected?
IX. What muscles attach to the coracoid process, and what nerves innervate them?
X. At what site is the clavicle most commonly fractured?
XI. In which direction are the resultant fragments displaced? Explain your answer.

Question 2

Scenario:
You are the surgical registrar on call. A young man is referred urgently, having been stabbed in his right axilla.

I. Define the boundaries of the axilla.
II. What major structures in the axilla could potentially be damaged?
III. To what structure are the cords of the brachial plexus intimately related?
IV. If the patient had been stabbed through the anterior aspect of his axilla, through what layers would the knife have passed to reach the structure mentioned in III?

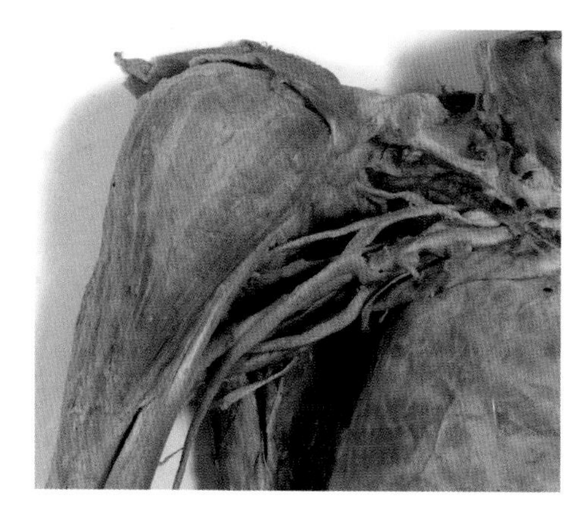

Image 1.2

With regards to Image 1.2:

V. Identify the structure referred to in III.
VI. Identify the medial and lateral cords of the brachial plexus.
VII. Name the branches of both of these cords.
VIII. Identify the major branches of the lateral cord in the above dissection.
IX. What are the root values of the musculocutaneous, median, ulnar, radial and axillary nerves?
X. Which muscles are supplied by the musculocutaneous nerve?
XI. What does the musculocutaneous nerve continue as?
XII. What clinical features would you expect if the musculocutaneous nerve was to be severed by this injury?

Question 3

Scenario:
A patient is complaining of pain on abduction of his shoulder.

I. What type of joint is the shoulder joint?
II. What factors contribute to the stability of the shoulder joint?
III. What muscles make up the rotator cuff, and what nerves innervate them?

(a)

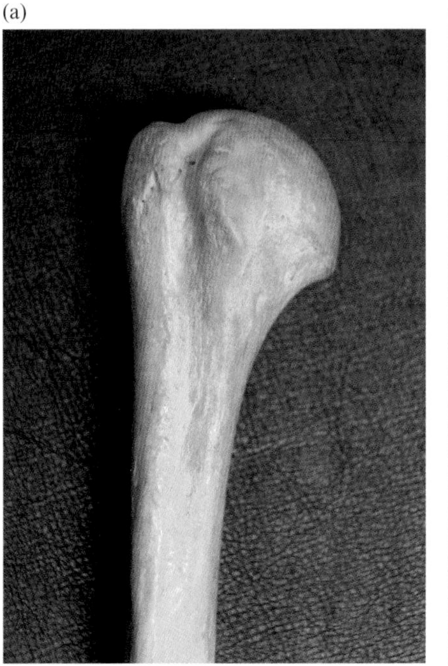

(b)

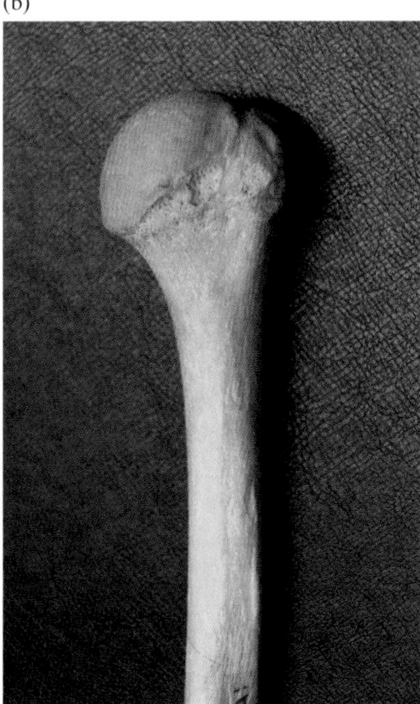

Image 1.3

With regards to Image 1.3:

IV. Using figure 1.3, demonstrate where each of the rotator cuff muscles insert.

V. On a colleague, demonstrate the following movements: flexion and extension, abduction and adduction, and internal and external rotation. What muscles are responsible for each action?
VI. On this same subject, isolate and test the function of the subscapularis muscle.
VII. Which nerve(s) innervates the serratus anterior muscle?
VIII. What are the consequences if this nerve is damaged?
IX. Demonstrate how you would test for a lesion of this nerve on a patient.

Question 4

Scenario:
You are in the accident and emergency (A&E) department teaching medical students how to perform an upper limb venepuncture and to take a radial artery blood gas sample.

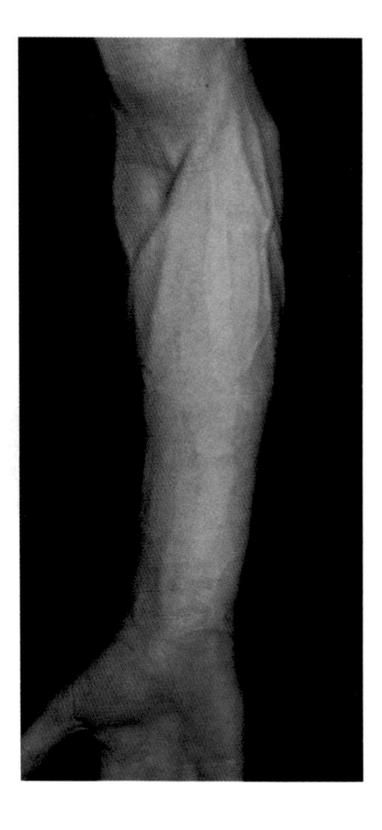

Image 1.4

With regards to Image 1.4:

I. Point to and name three vessels in this image that could be used for venepuncture.
II. What are the boundaries of the cubital fossa?
III. What major nerve could potentially be damaged when taking a sample of blood from a vein within the cubital fossa?
IV. Describe the functions of this nerve.
V. What examination can you perform prior to taking an arterial blood gas sample to assess the adequacy of the radial and ulnar arterial supply to the hand?

Whilst teaching the students, a patient is admitted having sustained hand trauma whilst operating machinery at work.

VI. Where do the tendons of the flexor digitorum profundus muscle insert?
VII. Where do the tendons of the flexor digitorum superficialis muscle insert?
VIII. How can you test the function of each of these two muscles?
IX. Is handgrip strongest when the wrist is flexed or extended? Explain the reason behind the answer.
X. What does the flexor tendon pulley system consist of?
XI. What are the contents of the carpal tunnel?
XII. What are the boundaries of the anatomical snuffbox?
XIII. What are the contents of the anatomical snuffbox?

Question 5

Scenario:
A patient from A&E who is complaining of a cold and pale foot is referred to you. The A&E officer is concerned that the patient has an acutely ischaemic foot. You are called to examine the patient's lower limb.

I. Describe the surface landmarks of the femoral artery.
II. Describe the surface landmarks of the dorsalis pedis artery.
III. Describe the surface landmarks of the posterior tibial artery.
IV. What structures run behind the medial malleolus?

You discover the patient has absent pulses distal to his femoral pulses. You decide to perform an ABPI examination.

V. What does ABPI stand for?
VI. How would you perform an ABPI examination?
VII. What ABPI result would contraindicate the use of thromboembolic deterrent (TED) stockings?

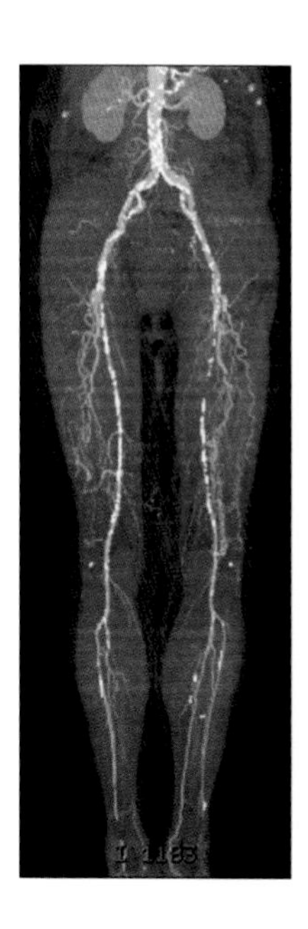

Image 1.5

VIII. In the angiogram shown in Image 1.5, which major artery is occluded?

With regards to the superficial venous drainage of the lower limb:

IX. What are the landmarks of the great (long) saphenous vein?

X. What nerve accompanies the great saphenous vein?

XI. What is the surface marking of the small (short) saphenous vein?

Question 6

Scenario:

A patient is admitted with a fractured neck of femur.

With regards to Image 1.6:

I. Identify the head.

II. Identify the neck.

III. Identify the greater trochanter.

IV. Identify the lesser trochanter.

V. Describe the blood supply to the head of the femur.

VI. Identify where the capsule of the hip joint is attached to the femur.

VII. What fused bones make up the pelvic girdle?

VIII. What factors maintain stability of the hip joint?

IX. What are the principal hip flexors?

X. What nerve(s) supply these muscles?

XI. Show the attachment of these muscles on Image 1.6.

XII. What muscles would you come across when performing a posterior approach to the hip?

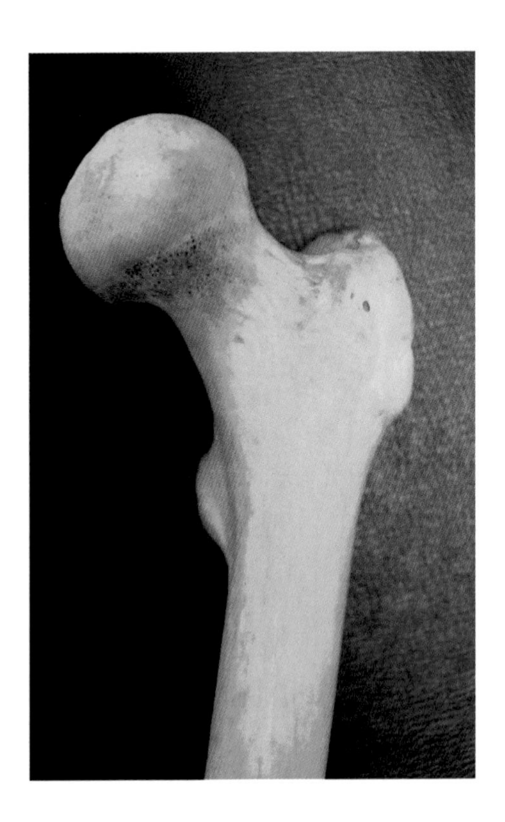

Image 1.6

XIII. What muscles attach to the greater trochanter?
XIV. What nerve supplies the two muscles attached to the greater trochanter arising from the ilium?
XV. What is their main function?
XVI. Demonstrate a clinical sign testing for the function of these muscles.
XVII. When would this test be positive?

Question 7

Scenario:
A patient presents with a lump in his popliteal fossa.

I. What are the boundaries of the popliteal fossa?

With regards to Image 1.7:

II. Identify the following structures:
   a. common fibular (peroneal) nerve
   b. tibial nerve
   c. popliteal vein
   d. popliteal artery.

III. What clinical effects are produced by an injury to the common fibular nerve?
IV. Identify the semitendinosus muscle.
V. Identify the medial head of the gastrocnemius muscle.
VI. What nerve innervates the gastrocnemius muscle?
VII. What is the function of the popliteus muscle?
VIII. Outline the lymphatic drainage of the lower limb.
IX. What is the differential diagnosis of a lump in the popliteal fossa?

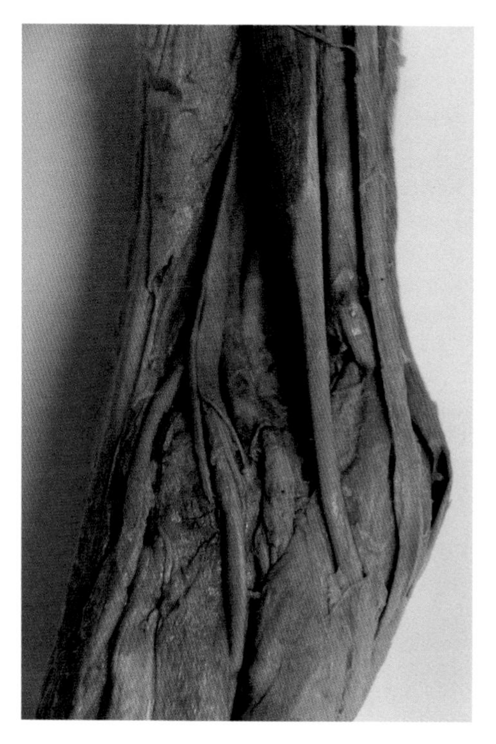

Image 1.7 **Left popliteal fossa**

Question 8

Scenario:
A patient complains of tingling, pain and numbness over the lateral aspect of his thigh.

I. What is a myotome?
II. What is a dermatome?

III. Demonstrate on a volunteer the dermatome distribution of the thigh.
IV. What cutaneous nerve innervates the lateral aspect of the thigh?
V. What condition may this patient be suffering from?
VI. What is the principal motor nerve of the anterior compartment of the thigh?
VII. What is the relationship of the femoral nerve to the femoral artery in the femoral triangle?
VIII. What are the boundaries of the femoral triangle?
IX. What are the contents of the femoral triangle?

Question 9

Scenario:
A patient presents to A&E following an injury to his knee, which he sustained during a basketball game.

I. What group of muscles are the principal flexors of the knee, and what nerve supplies these muscles?
II. If this nerve is damaged can the knee still be flexed?

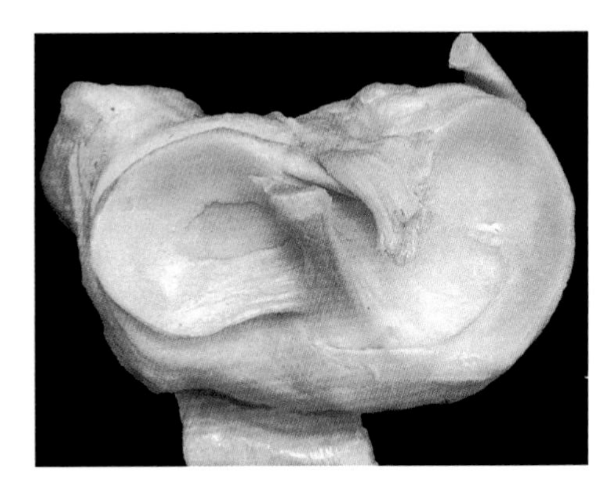

Image 1.8

With regards to Image 1.8:

III. Identify the posterior cruciate ligament.
IV. Identify the anterior cruciate ligament.
V. Identify the lateral meniscus.
VI. Identify the medial meniscus.

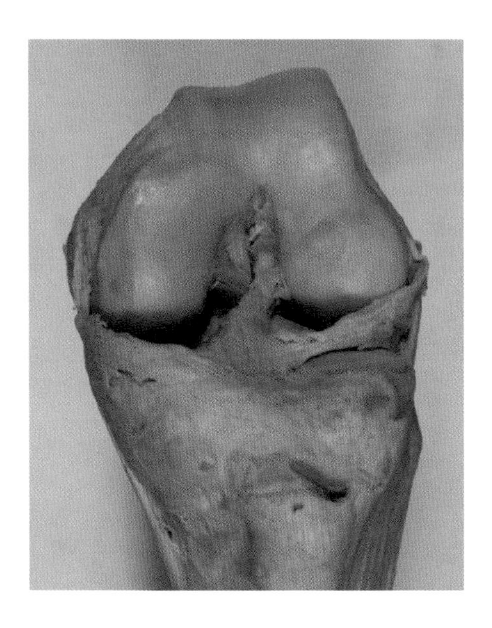

Image 1.9

With regards to Image 1.9:

VII. Identify the posterior cruciate ligament.
VIII. Identify the anterior cruciate ligament.
IX. Identify the lateral meniscus.
X. Identify the medial meniscus.
XI. What prevents the patella from migrating laterally?

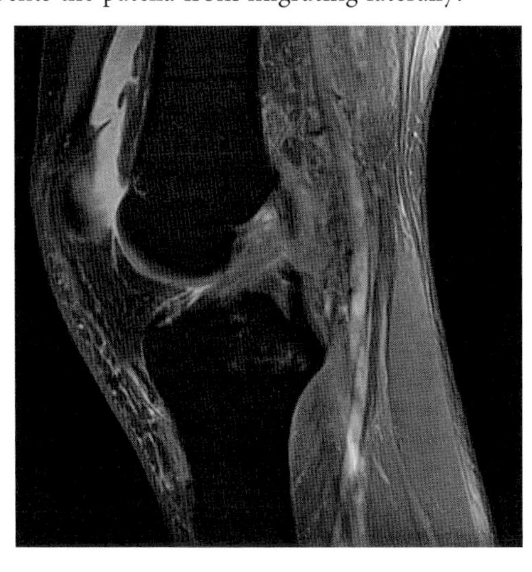

Image 1.10

With regards to Image 1.10:

XII. What pathology is shown in the MRI scan?
XIII. In what plane is this MRI scan displayed?

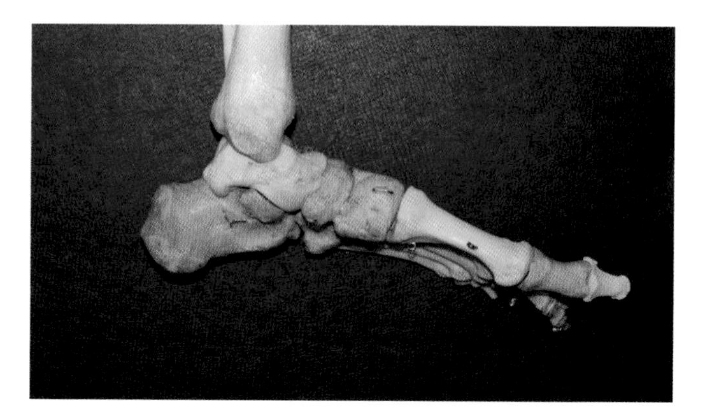

Image 1.11

With regards to Image 1.11:

XIV. Identify the medial malleolus.
XV. Identify the site of attachment of the deltoid ligament.
XVI. What muscles are responsible for everting and inverting the ankle?
XVII. What muscles are responsible for dorsiflexing and plantarflexing the ankle?
XVIII. What is the root value of the ankle reflex?

Question 10

Scenario:
You are the on-call surgeon, and a patient is referred to you with a tibial shaft fracture following a high-energy injury. During the night he complains of unbearable pain in the affected leg, which is refractory to opiate analgesia.

I. What is the likely diagnosis, and what is the pathology behind the clinical picture?
II. How many compartments are there in the leg?
III. Name the muscles in each compartment.
IV. What nerves or arteries run within each compartment?
V. Where does the gastrocnemius muscle insert?

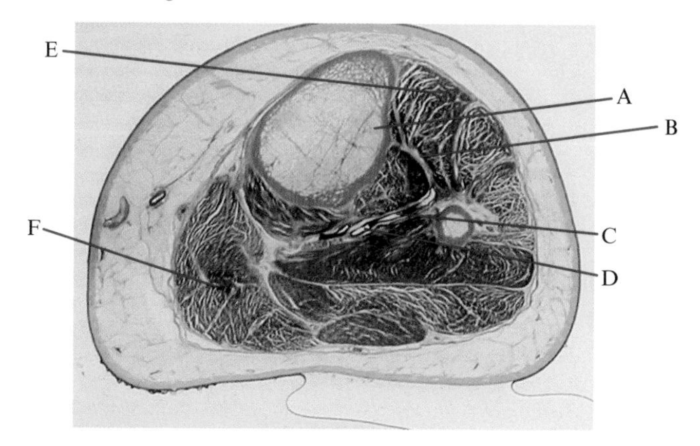

Image 1.12

With regards to Image 1.12:

VI. Identify all the compartments in the leg.
VII. What are the structures labelled A and B?
VIII. What are the structures labelled C and D?
IX. Identify muscle E and state its origins and action(s).
X. Identify muscle F and state its origins and action(s).

Question 11

Scenario:
A patient presents with back pain radiating down his leg.
With regards to Image 1.13:

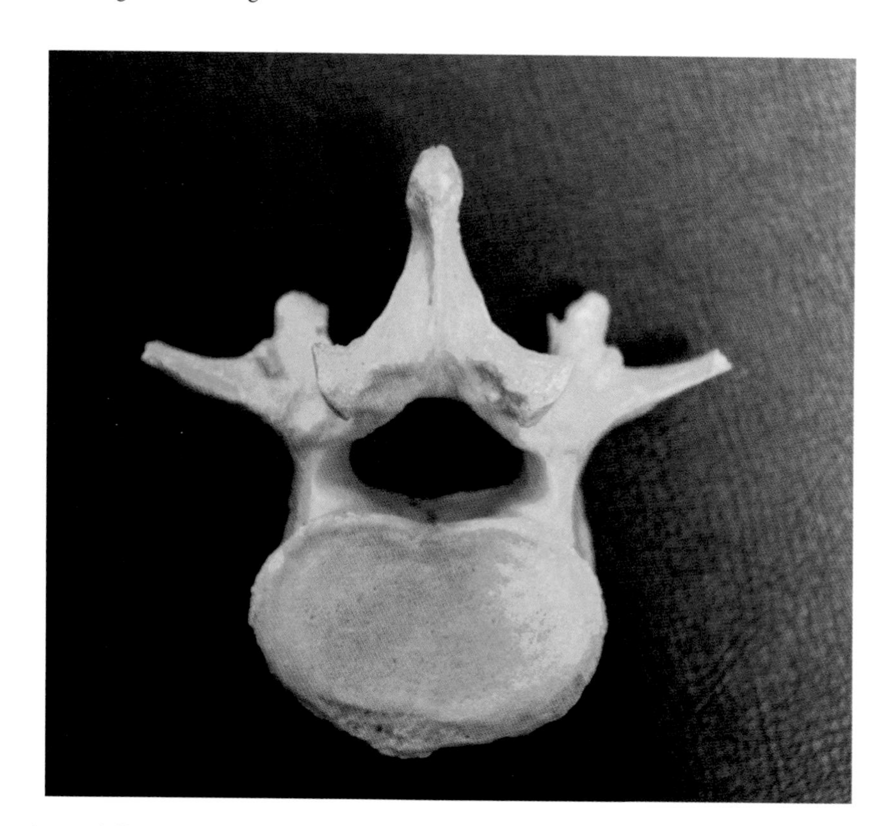

Image 1.13

I. Identify the body of this vertebra.
II. Identify the spine of this vertebra.
III. Identify the pedicles of this vertebra.
IV. What are the features of a typical cervical vertebra?
V. What type of joints are intervertebral joints?

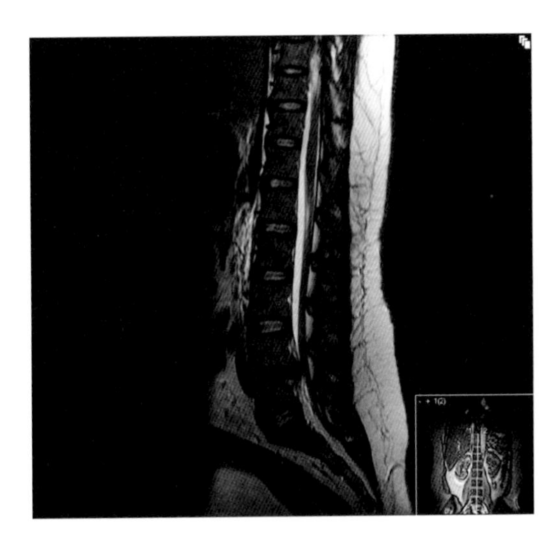

Image 1.14

VI. On the MRI scan in Image 1.14, identify the L3 vertebra.

With regards to Image 1.14:

VII. What pathology is shown in this scan?

VIII. What nerve root is likely to be affected by this pathology?

When performing a lumbar puncture, the relevant anatomy must be considered.

IX. At what level does the spinal cord end?

X. What layers or structures would the needle pass through when performing a lumbar puncture?

2

Limbs and vertebral column answers

Question 1

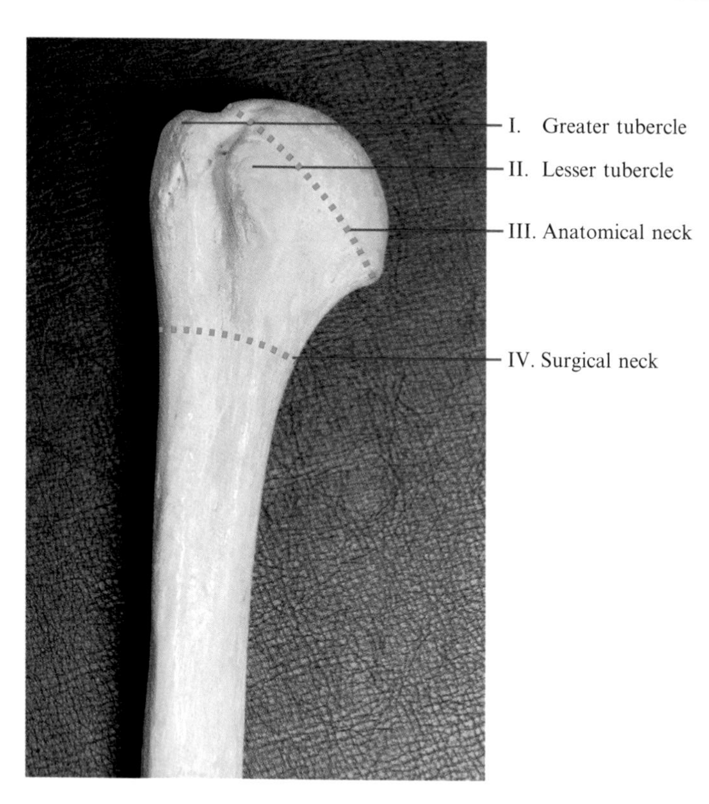

Image 2.1

I. The greater tubercle is the larger of the two tubercles and lies lateral to the lesser tubercle when the humerus is in the anatomical position; it projects lateral to the acromion. It has three facets, which provide attachment for three of the rotator cuff tendons (supraspinatus, infraspinatus and teres minor).

II. The lesser tubercle is smaller but still prominent. It is the site of attachment of the fourth rotator cuff tendon (subscapularis).

III. The anatomical neck of the humerus follows the articular margins of the head of the humerus. The capsule of the shoulder joint is attached to the anatomical neck, except medially and inferiorly where it attaches to the surgical neck of the humerus.

IV. The poorly defined surgical neck is at the upper end of the shaft of the humerus.

V. Fractures through the **surgical neck of the humerus** are the most common type of proximal humeral fracture. They are extracapsular and therefore rarely compromise the blood supply to the head of the humerus. Fractures of the anatomical neck of the humerus are rare. The **axillary nerve** (C5,6) passes immediately behind the surgical neck of the humerus, where it lies in contact with the bone just below the capsule of the shoulder joint. Consequently, it is susceptible to injury with fractures of the surgical neck and with shoulder dislocation.

VI. The axillary nerve is a branch of the posterior cord of the brachial plexus. It supplies motor innervation to the deltoid and teres minor muscles and sensory cutaneous supply to the upper lateral arm. Injury to the axillary nerve may result in the following signs:

- **Weakness** (and later wasting) of the deltoid muscle, causing a loss of power during abduction and later 'flattening' of the normally rounded contour of the shoulder.
- **Sensory loss** on the upper outer aspect of the arm, over the 'regimental patch' area.

The main differential diagnosis of an axillary nerve lesion is a C5 nerve root lesion. With the latter, the normal function of the suprascapular nerve (C5,6), which supplies the supraspinatus and infraspinatus muscles, will also be affected.

VII. The **radial nerve** (C5–8, T1). The radial nerve is the continuation of the posterior cord of the brachial plexus. It descends posterior to the axillary artery and enters the spiral (or radial) groove alongside the profunda brachii artery and its venae comitantes. It passes between the medial and long head of the triceps muscle and is in contact with the periosteum of the humerus in the lower part of the spiral groove.

VIII. In a fracture involving the spiral groove, the radial nerve could be injured, resulting in sensory and motor disturbances. Sensory impairment would be apparent in the territory supplied by the superficial radial nerve, but due to overlap of cutaneous innervation only a small area of anaesthesia would be evident, usually over the dorsum of the hand between the first and second metacarpal bones. This is therefore the autonomous zone and so the best area to test for sensory function of the radial nerve. Knowledge of where the motor branches leave the radial nerve can be used to predict the site of the lesion. The motor branches to the long and medial heads of the triceps leave the radial nerve proximal to the spiral groove; whereas the branch to the lateral head, and a second branch to the medial head, are generally given off more distally. Consequently, a fracture involving the spiral groove is likely to affect the lateral head with relative sparing of the long and medial heads. Elbow extension is weak rather than lost. Brachioradialis function will also be impaired. Both wrist and finger drop may be evident due to denervation of the wrist and long finger extensors, extensor pollicis longus and abductor pollicis longus. The interphalangeal joints of the fingers can still be extended due to the retained action of the intrinsic muscles of the hand.

IX. Three muscles attach to the coracoid process. They are the:
- **biceps brachii**, short head (musculocutaneous nerve);
- **coracobrachialis** (musculocutaneous nerve);
- **pectoralis minor** (medial and lateral pectoral nerves).

X. The clavicle is the most commonly fractured bone in the body. The junction between **middle and lateral thirds** is most commonly fractured (~75% of all clavicular fractures) for two reasons: (a) the medial two-thirds are circular in cross-section whilst the lateral third is flatter; the junction between the two regions is comparatively weak and also has no muscular attachments; (b) the powerful coracoclavicular and costoclavicular ligaments stabilise the lateral and medial third of the clavicle, respectively, and fractures therefore tend to occur between these points.

XI. The medial fragment of bone is elevated superiorly by the unopposed action of the sternocleidomastoid muscle. The lateral fragment is depressed by the weight of the arm. The proximal humerus may be pulled medially by the action of pectoralis major.

Question 2

I. The axilla is a pyramidal structure between the upper arm and upper outer thoracic wall. Its boundaries are as follows:
- **Apex** – communicates with the posterior triangle of the neck and is bounded by the clavicle, scapula and the outer border of the first rib.
- **Floor (base)** – axillary fascia (supported by the suspensory ligament) and skin.
- **Anterior wall** – pectoralis major and minor, and the clavipectoral fascia.
- **Posterior wall** – subscapularis, teres major and latissimus dorsi.
- **Medial wall** – the upper four ribs, their intercostal muscles and the upper part of serratus anterior.
- **Lateral** – the anterior and posterior walls converge on the intertubercular groove of the humerus.

II. This question is simply asking about the major contents of the axilla, which include:
- the **axillary vessels**, i.e. the axillary artery, vein and their branches/tributaries;
- the cords of the **brachial plexus** and their branches;
- **lymphatics**;
- **adipose tissue**;
- occasionally, the **axillary tail of the breast**.

III. The cords of the brachial plexus surround the **axillary artery**; they are named after their position relative to the second part of the artery (the part lying behind pectoralis minor).

IV. An anterior stab wound would penetrate:
- skin;
- subcutaneous fat;
- the fascia overlying pectoralis major and the muscle itself;
- the clavipectoral fascia and possibly pectoralis minor;
- the axillary sheath which surrounds the axillary artery.

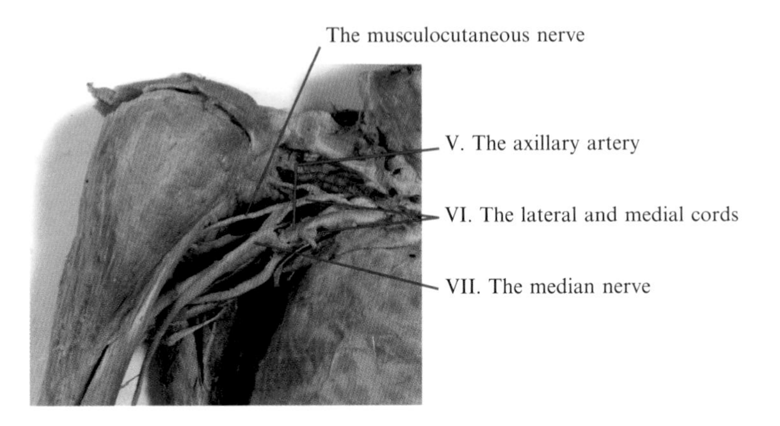

Image 2.2

V. The axillary artery can be seen in the dissection surrounded by the cords of the brachial plexus. Pectoralis minor has been removed.

VI. The lateral cord is formed from the anterior divisions of the upper and middle trunks; whereas the medial cord is a continuation of the anterior division of the lower trunk.

VII. The branches of the lateral cord are the **musculocutaneous nerve**, the **lateral pectoral nerve** and the lateral root of the **median nerve**. The medial cord contributes the other root to the **median nerve** and also gives off the **medial pectoral nerve, medial cutaneous nerve of the arm, medial cutaneous nerve of the forearm** and the **ulnar nerve**. The posterior cord typically has five branches (upper and lower subscapular nerves, thoracodorsal nerve, axillary nerve and radial nerve).

VIII. The musculocutaneous nerve arises from the lateral cord of the brachial plexus and passes laterally to pierce coracobrachialis, before descending between brachialis and biceps brachii. The median nerve originates on the lateral side of the third part of the axillary artery and, as it descends the arm, it crosses the brachial artery to lie on its medial side in the cubital fossa.

IX. The root value of the musculocutaneous nerve is **C5–7**. The median nerve has a root value of **C5–T1**, taking C5–7 from the lateral cord and C8, T1 from the medial cord. The ulnar nerve has a root value of **C7,8, T1;** the C7 fibres originating from a branch of the lateral cord, which is often not shown in diagrams of the brachial plexus. The radial nerve has a root value of **C5–8, T1**, and the axillary nerve has a root value of **C5,6.**

X. The musculocutaneous nerve supplies both heads of **biceps brachii**, **coracobrachialis** and most of **brachialis.**

XI. The musculocutaneous nerve continues as the **lateral cutaneous nerve of the forearm**, supplying skin over the radial side of the forearm.

XII. There would be **weakness** of elbow flexion and some **sensory impairment** over the anterolateral aspect of the forearm. There would not necessarily be complete sensory loss because of overlap of cutaneous nerves.

Question 3

I. The shoulder joint is a **typical synovial joint.** It is a multi-axial, ball-and-socket joint. The characteristics of a typical synovial joint are:
   a. enclosed within a capsule;
   b. non-articular surfaces lined by synovium;
   c. articulating bone ends covered by hyaline cartilage.

   If the articulating bone ends are covered by fibrocartilage instead of hyaline cartilage then the joint is known as an atypical synovial joint. Examples include the sternoclavicular and acromioclavicular joints.

II. The shoulder joint is inherently unstable (in order to maximise mobility), making it the most commonly dislocated joint in the body. Factors contributing to this instability include the fact that the glenoid fossa is shallow, the humeral head forms about one-third of a sphere, and the joint capsule being especially lax inferiorly. Numerous factors offset this instability, including the following:
   a. **Cartilage**: the glenoid labrum widens and deepens the glenoid fossa.
   b. **Intrinsic muscles**: the tendons of the rotator cuff muscles fuse with the lateral part of the joint capsule. These muscles maintain congruence between the humeral head and the glenoid fossa by applying compressive forces during shoulder movements.
   c. **Extrinsic muscles:** the long head of the biceps brachii attached to the supraglenoid tubercle of the scapula, and the long head of the triceps brachii attached to the inferior glenoid tubercle, provide support superiorly and inferiorly, respectively. This is particularly important when the shoulder is abducted.

d. **Ligaments:** the three glenohumeral ligaments (superior, middle and inferior) and the coracohumeral ligament strengthen the capsule. The superior glenohumeral and coracohumeral ligaments lie in the triangular gap between the supraspinatus and subscapularis tendons (the rotator interval). Together with the middle glenohumeral ligament they resist posterior and inferior instability. The inferior ligament (particularly its anterior band) is the primary restraint to anterior instability.

Other contributions are provided by the coracoacromial arch (coracoid process, acromion and the coracoacromial ligament) which helps protect from upward displacement, the deltoid muscle, and the negative intra-articular pressure.

An alternative but less detailed answer would be:

The glenohumeral joint is reliant on both **static** and **dynamic** stability.

- **Static** stability is provided by the head of the humerus fitting into the shallow glenoid fossa, reinforced by the surrounding glenoid labrum, the overlying joint capsule and the glenohumeral ligaments.
- **Dynamic** stability is provided by surrounding musculature, particularly the rotator cuff muscles, deltoid and the long head of the biceps (which lies within the shoulder joint having originated from the supraglenoid tubercle). Other contributory muscles include triceps, pectoralis major, latissimus dorsi and teres major.

III. The rotator cuff consists of four muscles:

- **supraspinatus** – suprascapular nerve (C5/6);
- **infraspinatus** – suprascapular nerve (C5/6);
- **subscapularis** – upper and lower subscapular nerves (C5/6);
- **teres minor** – axillary nerve (C5/6).

IV. Supraspinatus inserts into the highest facet of the greater tubercle. Its tendon passes under the coracoacromial ligament deep to the subacromial

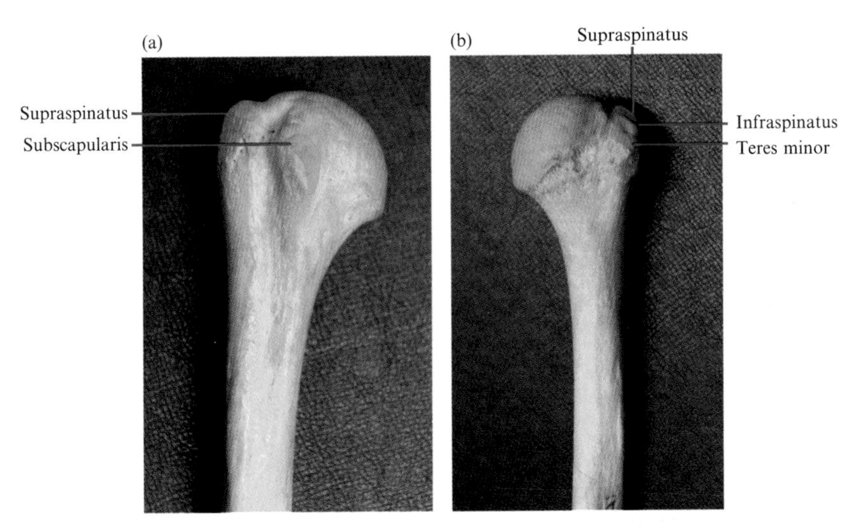

Image 2.3

bursa. The latter is continuous inferiorly with the subdeltoid bursa, together forming the largest bursa in the body. The tendon of supraspinatus may become inflamed in impingement syndromes.
Infraspinatus attaches to the middle facet of the greater tubercle, and teres minor to the lowest facet. Subscapularis inserts into the lesser tubercle, its tendon passing anterior to the capsule of the shoulder joint.

V. Since the glenoid fossa faces forwards and laterally with the upper limb relaxed at the side, the arm moves anteromedially in flexion and anterolaterally in abduction, but these movements are often described as occurring in the sagittal and coronal planes, respectively. The principle muscles involved in individual movements are as follows:
   - **Flexors** – pectoralis major, coracobrachialis, biceps and the anterior fibres of deltoid.
   - **Extensors** – teres major, latissimus dorsi and the posterior fibres of deltoid.
   - **Abduction** – deltoid, initially assisted by supraspinatus. The other three rotator cuff muscles counteract the strong upward pull of the deltoid muscle which would otherwise displace the humerus upwards. Abduction beyond about 90° is accompanied by lateral rotation of the humerus, and full abduction to 180° requires scapula rotation (principally by the trapezius and serratus anterior).
   - **Adduction** – pectoralis major and latissimus dorsi assisted by the rotator cuff muscles (except supraspinatus).
   - **Internal** (medial) rotation – pectoralis major, latissimus dorsi, teres major, the anterior fibres of deltoid and subscapularis.
   - **External** (lateral) rotation – infraspinatus, teres minor and the posterior fibres of deltoid.

VI. Subscapularis is principally an internal rotator and contributes to the formation of the posterior wall of the axilla. It can be tested by performing the **lift-off test:** place the subject's hand behind their back so that the dorsum of the hand is lying against the mid-lumbar spine. In this position, the shoulder is in maximal internal rotation and the action of pectoralis major is eliminated. Place your hand against the palmar aspect of the patient's hand and ask them to push against you. If a patient is unable to perform this manoeuvre they may have weakness in their subscapularis muscle.

VII. The **long thoracic nerve (of Bell[1])**. The root values are C5,6,7.

VIII. The patient may demonstrate **winging of the corresponding scapula**. They may complain of pain in the shoulder/scapular region and weakness performing tasks with the arms raised above the head.

IX. Winging of the scapula is best demonstrated by asking the patient to **push against resistance**, for example a door, with the elbow fully extended. This causes the medial border of the scapula to protrude from the back since it is no longer held against the ribs by serratus anterior.

Question 4

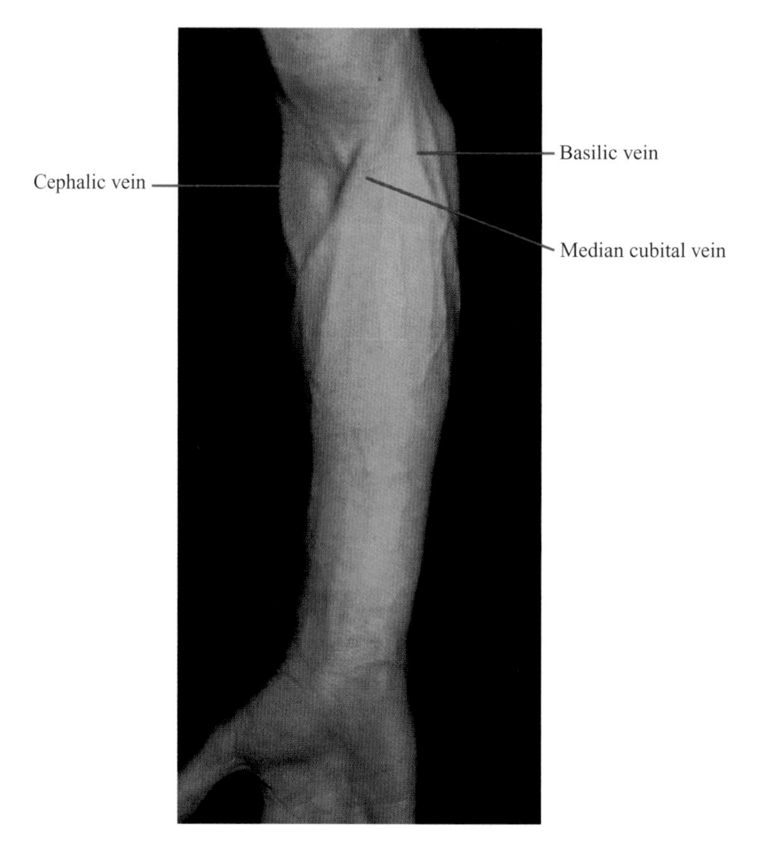

Image 2.4

I. The **cephalic**, **basilic** and **median cubital** veins are common sites for venepuncture.
   - The **cephalic vein** ascends on the lateral aspect of the upper limb within the superficial fascia to reach the deltopectoral groove, where it pierces the clavipectoral fascia to empty into the axillary vein.
   - The **basilic vein** ascends on the medial aspect of the upper limb also in the superficial fascia and perforates the deep fascia at mid-arm level to join the venae comitantes of the brachial artery, forming the axillary vein.
   - The **median cubital vein** is a prominent vein which joins the cephalic and basilic veins in a variable manner.

II. The **cubital fossa** is a triangular area on the anterior aspect of the elbow with the following boundaries:
   - superiorly – a line drawn between the medial and lateral epicondyles of the humerus;

- medially – the lateral border of pronator teres;
- laterally – the medial edge of brachioradialis;
- roof – formed by the deep fascia of the forearm, reinforced medially by the bicipital aponeurosis;
- floor – formed by the brachialis and supinator muscles.

III. The **median nerve** could potentially be damaged during venepuncture. The contents of the cubital fossa from medial to lateral are the:
- median nerve
- brachial artery with accompanying veins
- biceps tendon.

The radial nerve is sometimes also considered a content of the cubital fossa, but it actually lies just outside, under cover of brachioradialis.

IV. The median nerve has major sensory and motor functions in the forearm and hand.
- **Motor**: in the forearm, together with its anterior interosseous branch, it supplies all the muscles in the flexor compartment except for flexor carpi ulnaris and the ulnar half of flexor digitorum profundus. The median nerve enters the hand by passing through the carpal tunnel, giving off a recurrent (motor) branch which supplies the three thenar muscles (abductor pollicis brevis, flexor pollicis brevis and opponens pollicis) and motor branches to the first and second lumbrical muscles.
- **Sensory**: just proximal to the flexor retinaculum a palmar cutaneous branch is given off which supplies the skin over the thenar eminence. In approximately 20% of people the palmar cutaneous branch is given off distal to the flexor retinaculum. The palmar digital branches supply cutaneous sensation to the flexor surfaces and nailbeds of the radial three-and-a-half digits.

V. **Allen's test** is used to assess the blood supply to the hand and the adequacy of the individual ulnar and radial arteries. The test involves occluding both arteries by direct pressure, then exsanguinating the hand by asking the patient to lift their hand and repeatedly clench their fist until their hand turns pale. Pressure over the ulnar artery is then released and the colour should return rapidly to the hand, indicating that the ulnar artery is patent and capable of providing sufficient arterial flow to the hand if the radial artery flow was interrupted. If the hand is not reperfused within approximately 10 seconds, the radial artery should not be punctured or cannulated.

VI. The flexor digitorum profundus (FDP) tendons insert into the **bases of the distal phalanges**. The muscle originates from the proximal three-quarters of the ulnar and interosseous membrane. It is the only muscle which is able to flex the distal interphalangeal joints.

VII. The flexor digitorum superficialis (FDS) tendons insert into the **bodies of the middle phalanges**. The muscle has two heads. The humeroulnar head originates from the medial epicondyle of the humerus, the ulnar collateral ligament and the coronoid process of the ulnar. The radial head originates from the superior half of the anterior border of the radius.

VIII. The FDP muscle is tested by flexing the distal interphalangeal joint whilst holding the proximal joint in extension. The index finger may have independent function, but the remaining three fingers work together. Flexor digitorum superficialis has the ability to flex all the joints it passes. Furthermore it provides each finger with an individual slip whose function can be isolated. The FDS is tested by flexing a finger whilst the other three fingers are held in extension; this action isolates FDS from the action of FDP tendons.

IX. The flexors of the forearm, which are responsible for grip, are strongest when the wrist is in **extension**. This is because the tendons are stretched further and therefore providing a stronger contractile force.

X. The flexor tendon pulley system consists of the following structures:
- Five **annular** pulleys, numbered A1 to A5. The first or A1 pulley arises from the palmar plate of the metacarpophalangeal joint and the base of the proximal phalanx. It is released during treatment of stenosing tenosynovitis. The A2 pulley overlies the proximal phalanx and is the strongest. A3 is narrow and located anterior to the proximal interphalangeal joint. A4 overlies the middle phalanx and A5 overlies the distal interphalangeal joint. Surgically, the A2 and A4 pulleys are the most important for preventing bowstringing of the flexor tendons.
- Three **cruciate** pulleys, numbered C1 to C3. The C1 pulley lies just distal to the A2 pulley, the C2 pulley just distal to the A3 pulley, and the C3 pulley just distal to the A4 pulley.

The pulleys in the thumb are arranged differently.

XI. The carpal tunnel contains one nerve and nine tendons:
- median nerve – the most superficial structure in the tunnel;
- four tendons of FDS;

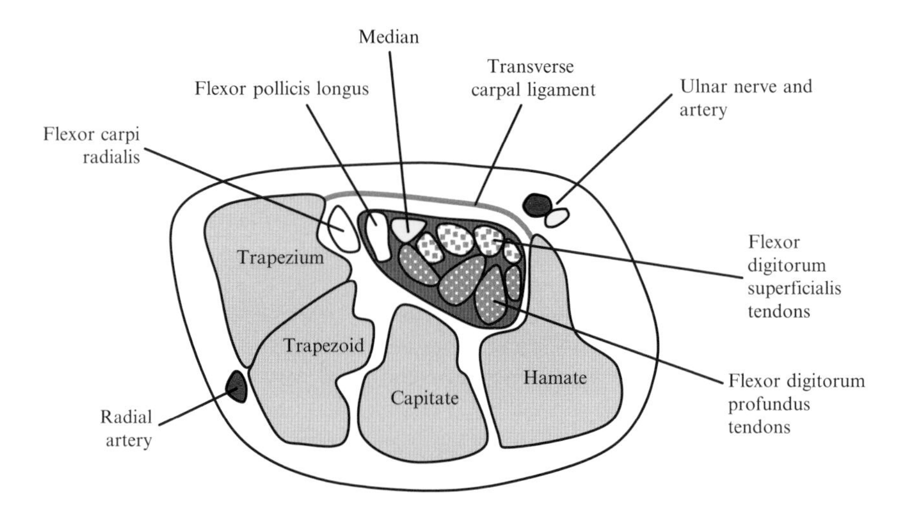

Image 2.5

- four tendons of FDP;
- the tendon of flexor pollicis longus.

The tendons of FDP and FDS are invested in a single synovial sheath, whilst flexor pollicis longus has its own separate synovial sheath.

XII. The boundaries of the anatomical snuffbox are as follows:
- anterior/radial border – the tendons of **abductor pollicis longus** and **extensor pollicis brevis**
- posterior or ulnar border – the tendon of **extensor pollicis longus**.

XIII. The contents of the anatomical snuffbox are as follows:
- The **radial artery**, which crosses the floor of the snuffbox deep to the tendons, forming its boundaries; a pulse is therefore palpable in the snuffbox.
- The **cephalic vein**, which originates from the dorsal veins of the hand in the snuffbox.
- The **radial styloid** and the **base of the first metacarpal**, which can be palpated in the floor of the snuffbox. The **scaphoid** and **trapezium** can be felt between the radial styloid and the base of the first metacarpal. Tenderness in the anatomical snuffbox may indicate a fracture of the scaphoid.

Question 5

I. The **femoral artery** begins as it passes below the inguinal ligament at the mid-inguinal point, which is midway between the anterior superior iliac spine and the pubic symphysis (note that this is different from the mid-point of the inguinal ligament which is midway between the anterior superior iliac spine and pubic tubercle). The femoral artery is known as the common femoral artery by vascular surgeons; it gives off the profunda femoris and continues as the superficial femoral artery along the proximal two-thirds of a line joining its origin with the adductor tubercle.

II. The **dorsalis pedis artery** is the continuation of the anterior tibial artery at the ankle, where it lies midway between the malleoli. It runs in the first intermetatarsal space and can be palpated against the tarsal bones just lateral to the tendon of extensor hallucis longus. Asking a patient to extend their toe may help you locate it. In approximately 10% of normal patients, the dorsalis pedis pulse may not be palpable.

III. The **posterior tibial artery** runs in the flexor compartment of the leg from the level of the neck of the fibula to a point midway between the medial malleolus and the Achilles tendon. The tibial nerve also runs along this line.

IV. From posterior to anterior, the tibialis posterior tendon, flexor digitorum longus tendon, posterior tibial artery, posterior tibial vein, tibial nerve and flexor hallucis longus tendon all run behind the medial malleolus. This can be remembered by the mnemonic 'Tom, Dick And Very Naughty Harry'.

V. The **Ankle Brachial Pressure Index** is a simple, non-invasive method of assessing the lower limb for arterial insufficiency. It is usually measured with a Doppler ultrasound probe and a sphygmomanometer (see below), comparing systolic pressure in the posterior tibial and dorsalis pedis arteries with that in the brachial artery. The ratio between the *systolic* blood pressure in the arm and leg estimates the severity of any arterial disease. The results can be interpreted as follows:

- >1 normal range;
- 0.4–0.9 peripheral arterial disease – this may be associated with intermittent claudication;
- 0–0.4 severe arterial disease which may be associated with rest pain and gangrene;
- >1.3 calcified, non-compressible vessels.

VI. Identify the brachial pulse with a Doppler probe. Place a sphygmomanometer cuff around the upper arm and inflate it until the Doppler signal is lost. Deflate the cuff and note the pressure at which the signal returns. Repeat the process on the other arm and use the highest value for calculating the ABPI. Perform the same procedure on the legs by placing a cuff above the medial malleolus and measure the pressures at the dorsalis pedis and posterior tibial pulses. Calculate the ABPI by dividing the highest ankle pressure by the highest brachial pressure.

VII. Thromboembolic deterrent stockings can be used safely when the ABPI is 0.8 and above, but are **contraindicated when the ABPI is below 0.5.** Between the two values, TED stockings may be used with caution, or antiembolism stockings with a reduced compression profile may be used instead.

VIII. The CT angiogram demonstrates a complete occlusion of the left **superficial femoral artery** with distal vessel reconstitution and good run off. The right superficial femoral artery is also diseased, but not occluded.

IX. The **great (long) saphenous vein** begins as the medial marginal vein of the foot. It is visible and palpable just anterior to the medial malleolus, from where it passes up the medial border of the tibia towards the knee, where it lies one hand's-breadth behind the medial border of the patella. It continues up the medial aspect of the thigh and enters the femoral vein at the saphenofemoral junction, which is 2.5–3.5 cm below and lateral to the pubic tubercle.

X. The great saphenous vein is accompanied by the **saphenous nerve** below the knee. The saphenous nerve is the largest cutaneous branch of the femoral nerve and supplies sensation to the medial side of the leg and foot.

XI. The small saphenous vein lies behind the medial malleolus (with the sural nerve), ascending in the subcutaneous fat behind the middle of the calf to the popliteal fossa. It enters the popliteal vein at a variable level.

Question 6

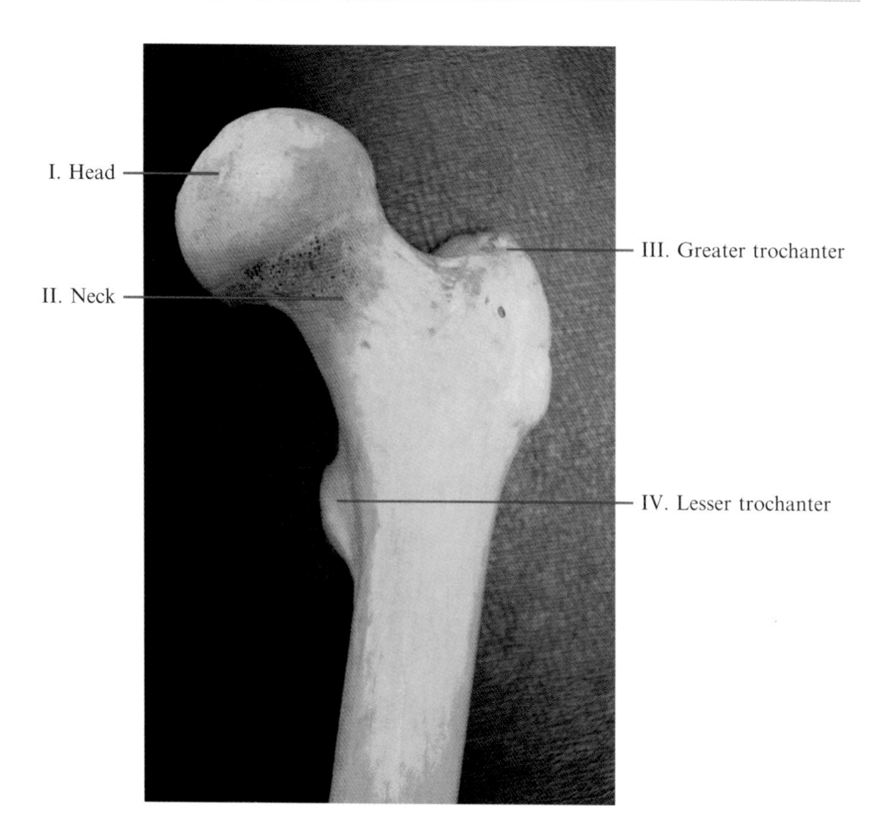

Image 2.6

I. The **femoral head** is intracapsular and surrounded by the acetabular labrum. The ligamentum teres attaches to the fovea. The head faces anteriorly, medially and superiorly.
II. The **femoral neck** is approximately 5 cm long. The neck shaft angle (or angle of inclination) is approximately 125°, and the neck is slightly anteverted, some 10–15°. Anteriorly, the neck is intracapsular, with the capsule attaching to the intertrochanteric line; however, posteriorly only the medial portion of the neck is intracapsular.
III. The **greater trochanter** can be palpated a hand's-breadth below the tubercle of the iliac crest and is in line with the femoral head.
IV. The **lesser trochanter** is a posteromedial projection from the shaft of the femur. The iliopsoas tendon attaches to it.
V. The head of the femur receives blood from the following sources:
   a. **Retinacular vessels**: the main blood supply originates from an extracapsular arterial ring, predominantly supplied by the medial and lateral

circumflex arteries, reinforced by the superior and inferior gluteal arteries. Ascending cervical branches enter the capsule beneath the synovial membrane, forming the retinacular arteries, the most significant of which lie posterior to the femoral neck. The retinacular vessels give rise to a subsynovial intracapsular arterial ring, which supplies both the epiphysis and metaphysis.

b. **Artery of the ligamentum teres**: an artery within the ligamentum supplies the epiphysis with a small amount of blood, particularly in young children. This artery is derived from the medial circumflex femoral artery and the obturator artery.

c. **Metaphyseal vessels**: after fusion of the epiphysis, metaphyseal arteries also contribute to the blood supply of the head of the femur, but this is not a major source of blood.

VI. The hip joint capsule encloses the hip joint and most of the neck of the femur. Anteriorly the capsule is attached to the **intertrochanteric line**. Posteriorly it is attached to the neck, approximately **1 cm medial** to the **intertrochanteric crest**.

VII. The pelvis or innominate bone is made up of three individual bones: the **ilium**, **ischium** and **pubis**. They meet at the acetabulum where they are separated by the tri-radiate cartilage (Y shaped), which ossifies at about 16–18 years of age.

- **Ilium**: the ilium makes up the superior two-fifths of the acetabulum, where it fuses with the pubis and the ischium. It expands above, forming the smooth concavity of the false pelvis above the pelvic brim, together with the iliac crest, which is an important region for abdominal and lower limb muscle attachment.
- **Pubis**: the body of the pubis forms the medial portion of the innominate bone and connects with the adjacent pubis at the pubic symphysis. From the body of the pubis, two rami extend. The superior pubic ramus extends up and back to form the anterior aspect of the acetabulum. The inferior pubic ramus extends down and laterally to join the ischial ramus, the site of attachment of the adductor muscles, making up the inferomedial border of the obturator foramen.
- **Ischium**: the body of the ischium forms the posteroinferior aspect of the acetabulum. The ischial spine projects from the body and gives attachment to the sacrospinous ligament, which separates the greater and lesser sciatic foramina. The ischial tuberosity forms the lateral boundary of the pelvic outlet and is the portion of the innominate bone on which we sit.

VIII. The hip joint is a multi-axial, synovial, ball-and-socket joint. It is very stable and requires considerable force to dislocate it. As with any joint, the stability of the hip joint is maintained by several factors:

a. **Bones**: the hip joint consists of the femoral head (slightly more than half a sphere), which articulates with the cup-shaped (cotyloid) acetabulum. This acetabular fossa is deepened by the acetabular labrum, a fibrocartilaginous rim that helps keep the femoral head in the acetabular socket. The joint has a negative pressure, causing a vacuum-like effect.

b. **Joint capsule**: the capsule is a dense structure attached to the acetabulum, to the inter-trochanteric line, and just medial to the inter-trochanteric crest enclosing the femoral head and neck. It is thickest anterosuperiorly, the area of maximal stress, and thin and more loosely attached posteroinferiorly.

c. **Ligaments**: three major ligaments reinforce the joint capsule. The strongest is the *iliofemoral ligament*, an inverted Y-shaped ligament anterior to the joint capsule. The *pubofemoral ligament* is deep to the medial component of the iliofemoral ligament and attaches to the superior pubic ramus and adjacent areas. The *ischiofemoral ligament* is located on the posterior aspect of the capsule, embracing the femoral neck. Two further ligaments are present: the transverse acetabular ligament, which bridges the acetabular notch and is continuous with the acetabular labrum; and the ligamentum teres, which tightens when the thigh is semi-flexed and adducted.

d. **Muscles**: several groups of muscles connect the pelvis to the femur, providing both movement and stability. Muscular action and tone are a major component of hip joint stability.

IX. The **psoas major** and **iliacus** muscles are the principal hip flexors. Other muscles which contribute include pectineus, rectus femoris, adductor longus and sartorius.

X. Psoas major is supplied by the ventral rami of **L1 and L2** spinal nerves, with a small contribution from L3. Iliacus is innervated by the **femoral nerve** (L2–4).

XI. Iliacus and psoas major join to form a common tendon (iliopsoas tendon) which inserts into the **lesser trochanter** of the femur (see Image 2.6). Iliacus originates from the superior two-thirds of the iliac fossa, iliac crest, the lateral sacrum and the ventral sacroiliac ligaments. Psoas major originates from the transverse processes, bodies and intervertebral discs of the lumbar vertebrae (lower border T12 to upper border of L5). It converges with the ipsilateral iliacus muscle before passing to the lesser trochanter.

XII. The posterior hip approach involves a lateral incision over the greater trochanter in line with the femur. The fascia lata is divided and the gluteus maximus and medius muscles exposed and split in the line of their fibres. The short external rotators are divided at their femoral attachments (piriformis, obturator internus and the gemelli, quadratus femoris) and the sciatic nerve is retracted medially and covered by the cut ends of the obturator internus and gemelli muscles, exposing the hip joint capsule.

XIII. There are many muscles attached to the greater trochanter:
- gluteus medius and minimus
- piriformis
- obturator internus and the gemelli
- obturator externus (trochanteric fossa)
- quadratus femoris (to the quadrate tubercle on the intertrochanteric crest)
- vastus lateralis.

XIV. Gluteus medius and minimus are innervated by the **superior gluteal nerve** (L4, L5, S1).

XV. Gluteus medius and minimus **abduct the thigh**; they also act as medial rotators. This action is particularly important when the contralateral leg is lifted off the ground when walking – the gluteus medius and minimus on the planted foot contract forcefully to prevent the pelvis tilting to the side of the lifted leg. In doing so, the lifted foot is raised higher than the planted foot.

XVI. **Trendelenburg's sign**[2] tests the strength of the hip abductors. The patient is asked to stand on one leg and the pelvis on the opposite side should rise slightly as a result of activation of the abductors on the side of the planted foot. If the pelvis on the side of the unsupported leg dips below that of the planted leg due to weakness of the hip abductor muscles, the Trendelenburg sign is positive. Note the difference between Trendelenburg's sign and test – the Trendelenburg test assesses the competency of valves in the superficial veins of the lower limb.

XVII. Trendelenburg's sign is positive when there is **weakness of the hip abductor muscles**. Causes include:
- paralysis of the gluteus medius and minimus
- congenital dislocation of the hip
- coxa vara.

The sign can be falsely positive if the patient has hip pain, e.g. in osteoarthritis of the hip.

Question 7

I. The **popliteal fossa** is diamond shaped with the following boundaries:
Superolateral – biceps femoris.
Superomedial – semimembranosus with overlying semitendinosus.
Inferolateral – lateral head of gastrocnemius with underlying plantaris.
Inferomedial – medial head of gastrocnemius.
Floor (anterior surface) – the posterior surfaces of the femur and tibia, the oblique popliteal ligament reinforcing the capsule of the knee joint and the popliteus muscle.
Roof (posterior surface) – popliteal fascia, pierced by the small (short) saphenous vein and the accompanying sural nerve.

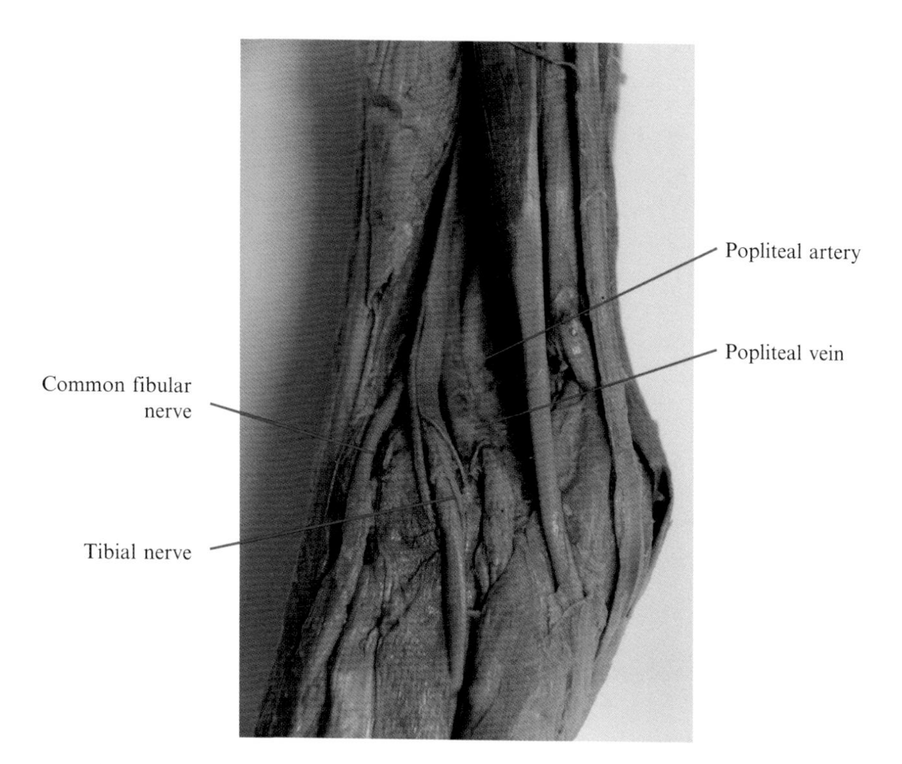

Image 2.7a

II. See Image 2.7a.

Note that the nerves are most superficial.

a. The common fibular nerve runs along the medial border of biceps femoris and leaves the popliteal fossa by passing over the lateral head of gastrocnemius, medial to the biceps tendon, from where it winds around the neck of the fibula into the substance of peroneus longus.

b. The tibial nerve passes vertically down the middle of the fossa and passes between the heads of gastrocnemius. It gives off branches to gastrocnemius, soleus, plantaris and popliteus. It also gives off the *sural nerve* which is joined by the sural communicating nerve (a branch of the common fibular nerve); the sural nerve runs adjacent to the small saphenous vein. The popliteal vessels lie deep to the nerves and are enclosed in a fibrous sheath.

c. The popliteal vein is superficial to the artery and receives the small saphenous vein in its course.

d. The popliteal artery is the deepest of the neurovascular structures. It divides into anterior and posterior tibial arteries at the inferior border of popliteus. It has five named genicular branches which supply the knee joint and surrounding muscles.

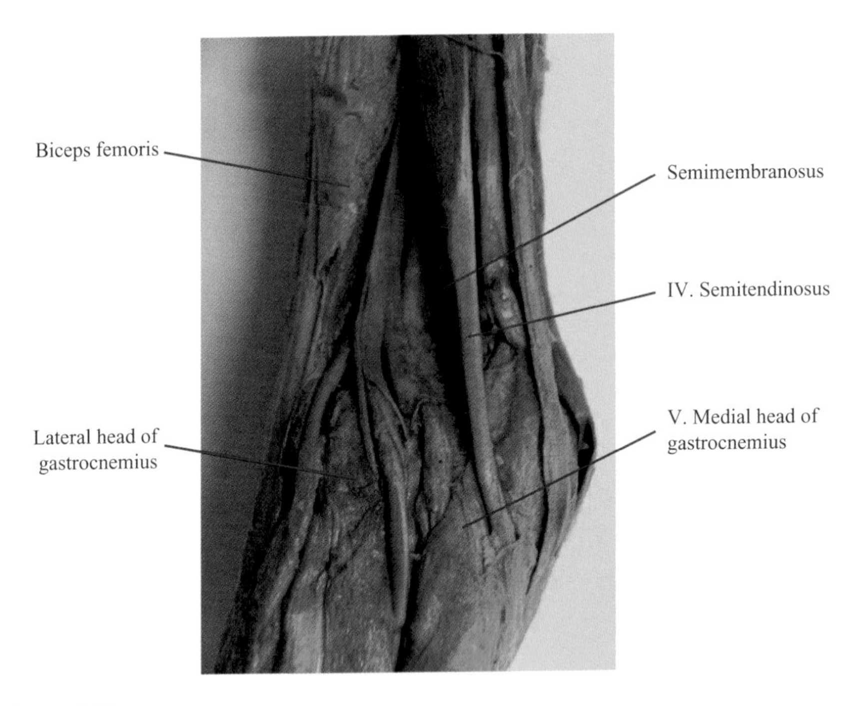

Image 2.7b

III. Injury to the common fibular nerve will cause the following:
- **Foot drop** due to weakness of dorsiflexion (anterior compartment, deep fibular nerve).
- **Weakness of eversion** (lateral compartment, superficial fibular nerve).
- **Weakness of toe extension** (extensor hallucis longus, deep peroneal nerve).
- **Sensory loss** over the lower lateral leg and dorsum of the foot; the most autonomous area for examination being the first dorsal web space, innervated by the deep branch of the nerve.

As a compensatory mechanism, a patient may adopt a high stepping gait. The common fibular nerve is particularly at risk of injury as it winds around the neck of the fibula, where it may be compressed e.g. by plaster casts or operating table supports. It may also be injured following fractures to the fibula or following knee injuries causing traction on the nerve.

IV. Note the difference between the semimembranosus, which has a long, flat, proximal ('membranous') tendinous origin from the ischial tuberosity, and semitendinosus, which has a long, cord-like tendon that inserts into the pes anserinus (goose's foot) of the tibia.

V. Gastrocnemius is the most superficial muscle of the posterior (flexor) compartment of the leg. The medial head is the larger of the two. Rarely, a third (popliteal) head may be present.

VI. Gastrocnemius is innervated by the **tibial nerve** (S1,2).

VII. Popliteus **'unlocks' the knee** by rotating the tibia medially on the femur or, if the foot is planted, rotating the femur laterally on the tibia.

VIII. The lymphatic drainage of the lower limb accompanies the venous drainage and so is divided into superficial and deep pathways. Superficial lymphatics accompany the saphenous veins. Those accompanying the great saphenous vein enter the superficial inguinal lymph nodes and ultimately drain into the external iliac lymph nodes. Lymphatics accompanying the small saphenous vein drain to popliteal nodes. The deep lymphatic vessels of the leg also enter the popliteal nodes, whose efferent vessels ultimately drain to deep inguinal nodes via lymphatics accompanying the femoral vessels. Lymphadenopathy should therefore be assessed by palpating the popliteal fossa and femoral triangle.

IX. When answering such a question, it is important to structure your answer. A simple way of doing so is in tissue structures, layer by layer. However it is important to try to list your differential diagnoses in order of their relative frequency. The differential diagnosis would include:
- venous – deep vein thrombosis or varicosities;
- arterial – popliteal artery aneurysm;
- lymphatic – lymphadenopathy (particularly from lesions on the lateral aspect of the leg and heel);
- joint/bursae – Baker's cyst[3] (usually a swelling of the gastrocnemius or semimembranosus bursa) or knee joint effusion;
- bone – bone tumours arising from the distal femur or proximal tibia;
- skin/subcutaneous tissue – sebaceous cyst/lipoma;
- neural – neurofibroma.

Question 8

I. A myotome is **the muscle territory supplied by a single segment of the spinal cord.**

II. A dermatome is **the area of skin supplied by a single spinal nerve, via both its rami.**

III. The anterior, medial and lateral aspects of the thigh are supplied by L1 to L3 (see Image 2.8). The L1 nerve root innervates the area of the groin crease (overlapping with T12) and the anterior region of the genitalia. The L2 nerve root supplies most of the lateral aspect of the upper thigh, and the L3 nerve root supplies most of the medial and inferior aspect of the thigh, including the skin over the knee. The posterior aspect of the thigh is supplied mostly by the S1 and S2 nerve roots.

IV. The lateral aspect of the thigh is innervated by the **lateral cutaneous nerve of the thigh**, whose sensory nerve roots must therefore be L2 and L3; it is a branch of the lumbosacral plexus.

V. **Meralgia paraesthetica**. The lateral cutaneous nerve of the thigh may become trapped as it descends under or through the inguinal ligament, medial to the anterior superior iliac spine. This causes altered sensation, paraesthesiae and pain in its sensory distribution.

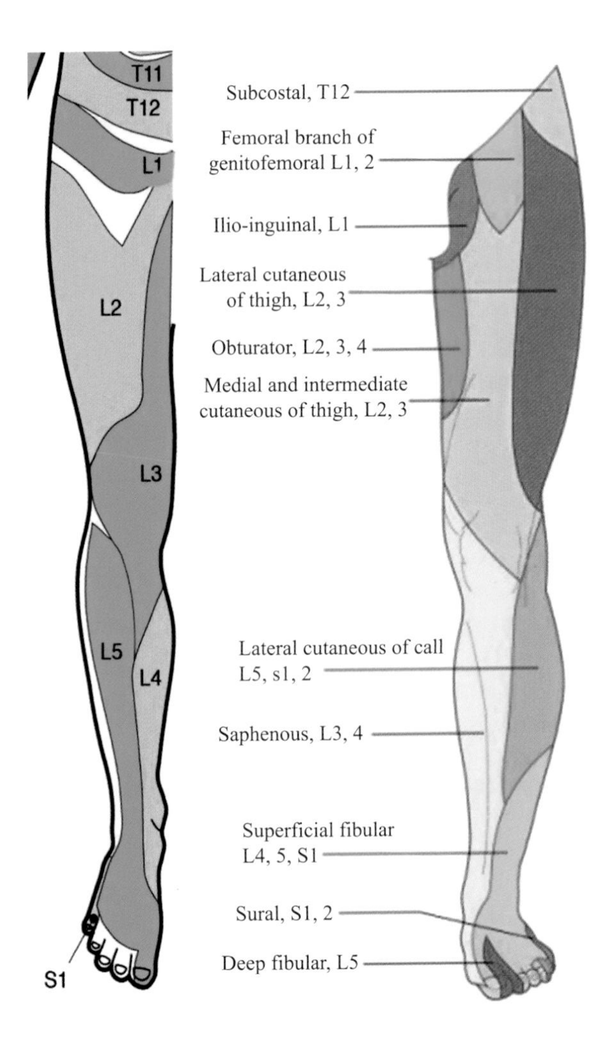

Image 2.8

VI. The **femoral nerve** supplies the anterior compartment of the thigh, the muscles of which are principally knee extensors, but also flex, rotate and adduct the hip. The femoral nerve is the largest branch of the lumbosacral plexus and has a root value of L2–4. Its terminal branch is the saphenous nerve.

VII. The femoral nerve lies **lateral to the femoral artery** in the femoral triangle.

VIII. The femoral triangle is a depressed intermuscular area on the front of the thigh immediately below the inguinal ligament (see Image 2.9). It consists of an inverted triangle with the following boundaries:

- **base** – the inguinal ligament
- **apex** – where sartorius overrides adductor longus

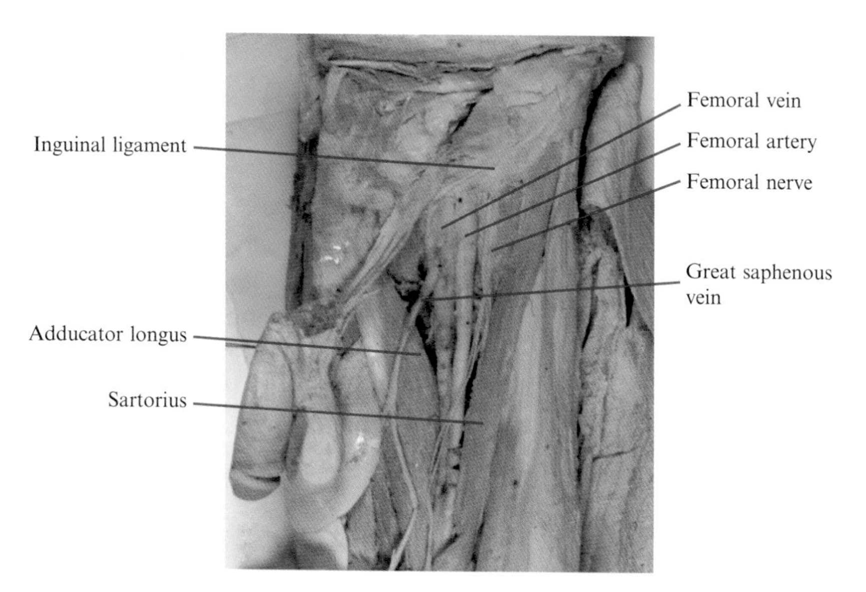

Image 2.9

- **medial border** – the *medial* border of adductor longus
- **lateral border** – the *medial* border of sartorius
- **floor** – from lateral to medial: iliacus, psoas, pectineus and adductor longus muscles
- **roof** – the fascia lata.

IX. The contents of the femoral triangle, from lateral to medial are the following:
- **The femoral nerve** (outside the femoral sheath).
- The femoral sheath, containing the **femoral artery** laterally, the **femoral vein** and, most medially, the **femoral canal**. The femoral canal contains lymphatics and fat and is the site of a femoral hernia.
- For the purists, the femoral branch of the genitofemoral nerve is also a transient content of the femoral sheath. The great saphenous vein joins the femoral vein in the femoral triangle by piercing the cribriform fascia overlying the saphenofemoral junction (see Question 5, part IX for the surface marking of this junction).

Question 9

I. The **hamstring muscles** are the principal knee flexors. They are innervated by the **sciatic nerve** and comprise the following muscles:
- semitendinosus (tibial nerve)
- semimembranosus (tibial nerve)

- biceps femoris (long head – tibial nerve; short head – common fibular nerve).

II. Yes. The pes anserinus (Latin for goose's foot) is the common attachment site of three muscles – sartorius, gracilis and semitendinosus. Sartorius and gracilis are innervated by the femoral and obturator nerves, respectively. Sartorius and gracilis are weak flexors of the knee, and therefore the knee can still be flexed when there is a sciatic nerve injury.

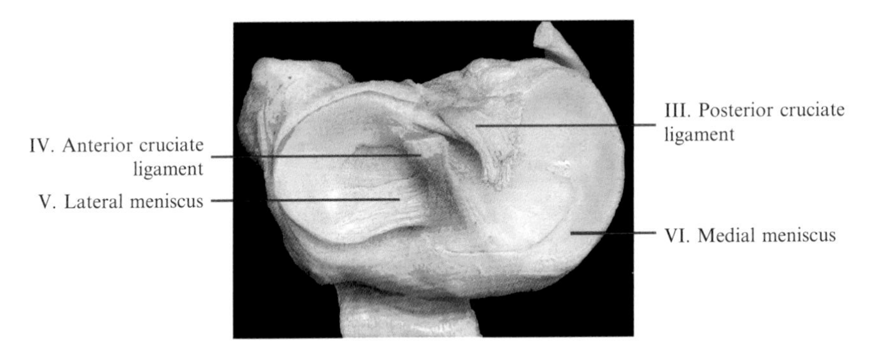

Image 2.10

III. The **posterior cruciate ligament** (PCL), the stronger of the two cruciate ligaments, is attached to the **posterior intercondylar area** of the tibia and an adjacent depression on the posterior surface of the tibia, passing superiorly, anteriorly and medially, to attach to the lateral surface of the medial femoral condyle. In simple terms, the PCL is taut during knee flexion and prevents posterior displacement of the tibia on the femur.

IV. The **anterior cruciate ligament** (ACL) is attached to the **anterior intercondylar area** of the tibia, where its fibres blend with the anterior horn of the lateral meniscus. It ascends superiorly, posteriorly and laterally to insert into the posteromedial aspect of the **lateral femoral condyle.** Again, simplifying its function, the ACL is taut when the knee is in extension, preventing hyperextension and anterior displacement of the tibia on the femur.

V. The **lateral meniscus** forms four-fifths of a circle. The anterior horn is attached just posterolateral to the anterior cruciate ligament. There is a gap between it and the lateral collateral ligament through which the popliteus tendon runs. The posterior horn of the lateral meniscus is connected to the medial femoral condyle via the meniscofemoral ligament(s).

VI. The **medial meniscus** forms a C-shape. Its anterior horn is attached to the anterior intercondylar area, just anterior to the origin of the ACL. Its posterior horn is attached to the posterior intercondylar area, between the posterior horn of the lateral meniscus and the PCL. Functions of the menisci include contributing to joint stability and congruity, load transmission, acting as shock absorbers, reducing contact stresses and proprioception.

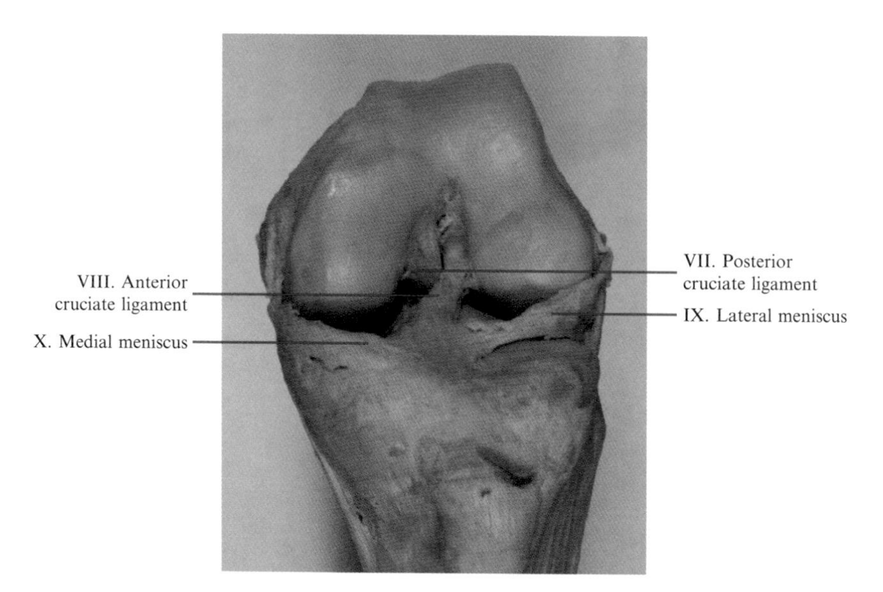

Image 2.11

VII. See Image 2.11.
VIII. See Image 2.11.
IX. See Image 2.11.
X. See Image 2.11.
XI. The patella is a sesamoid bone which articulates with the patellar surface of the femur. Lateral migration is prevented by:
- the distal insertion of **vastus medialis** muscle fibres into the patella;
- attachment of the **patellar retinacula** to the collateral ligaments;
- the anterior projection of the **lateral femoral condyle**, which provides bony resistance.

XII. The MRI scan shows an **ACL rupture** (see Image 2.12). The ACL fibres are indistinct and disrupted, consistent with a complete tear. There is also a small joint effusion.
Anterior cruciate ligament injuries generally occur when the foot is planted and the knee is subjected to a twisting motion. Meniscal tears are associated with 50–70% of acute ACL ruptures. The lateral meniscus is the most commonly affected with the initial injury; however the presence of a haemarthrosis offers a good environment for the lateral meniscus to heal. The abnormal loading and shear stresses in an anterior-cruciate-deficient knee may later lead to a tear of the medial meniscus, owing to its firm attachment to the joint capsule.

XIII. This is a **sagittal image**; i.e. a plane parallel to the median plane of the body.

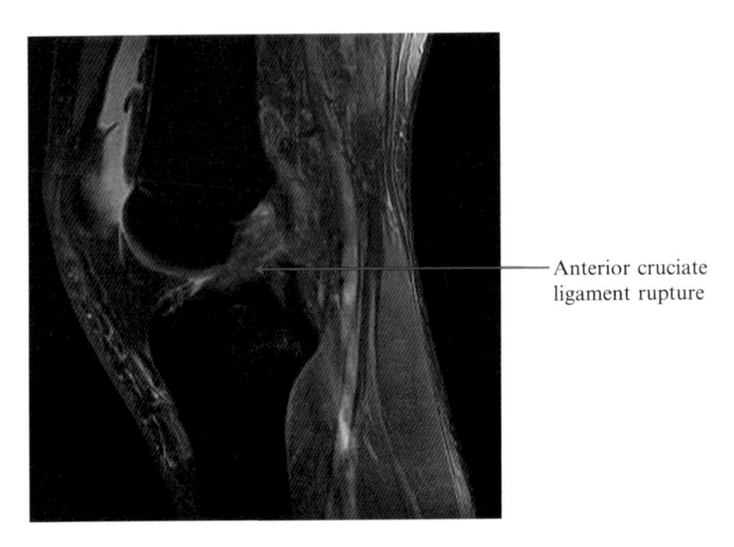

Image 2.12

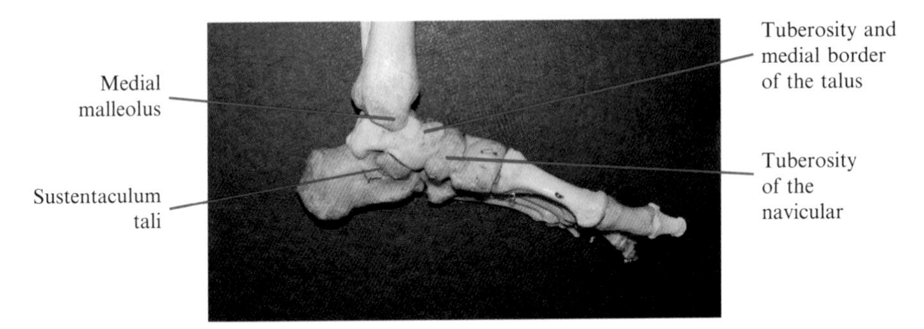

Image 2.13

XIV. The **medial malleolus** articulates with the medial surface of the talus. It ends more proximally and anteriorly than the lateral malleolus. Attached to it are the ankle joint capsule, the deltoid ligament, the flexor retinaculum and the inferior extensor retinaculum.

XV. The **deltoid** or medial collateral ligament is a complicated ligament that originates from the medial malleolus. It fans out in a triangular shape with superficial and deep fibres. The superficial fibres attach to the following structures:
- the tuberosity of the **navicular bone**;
- the **sustentaculum tali** (a projection from the medial side of the calcaneus);
- the medial border and medial tubercle of the **talus**;
- the medial margin of the **plantar calcaneo-navicular** (spring) ligament.

The deep fibres insert into:
- the non-articular surface of the medial talus.

This ligament is rarely injured except in association with fractures of the ankle joint.

XVI. Ankle eversion and inversion are brought about by movement at the *subtalar joint.*
Eversion is produced by contraction of the following muscles:
- **peroneus longus** (superficial fibular nerve)
- **peroneus brevis** (superficial fibular nerve)
- **peroneus tertius** (deep fibular nerve).

Inversion is produced by contraction of the following muscles:
- **tibialis anterior** (deep fibular nerve)
- **tibialis posterior** (tibial nerve).

XVII. Dorsiflexion and plantarflexion are the result of movement at the ankle (*talocrural*) joint. Dorsiflexion is produced mainly by muscles in the anterior compartment of the leg, which are innervated by the deep fibular nerve. The responsible muscles are:
- **tibialis anterior** (through which the majority of the force is produced)
- **extensor hallucis longus**
- **extensor digitorum longus**
- **peroneus tertius.**

Plantar flexion is brought about mainly through the Achilles (calcaneal) tendon, which is the common tendon of the superficial posterior group of calf muscles. However, the deep posterior group of muscles also contribute to plantar flexion. The tibial nerve supplies both groups, which consist of the following muscles:
- superficial group – **gastrocnemius**, **soleus** and **plantaris**
- deep group – **tibialis posterior**, **flexor hallucis longus** and **flexor digitorum longus.**

XVIII. **S1,2.** This is a commonly asked question and so you should remember the nerve root values of all the reflexes in the body. The other important lower limb reflex is the knee, which is L2–4.

Question 10

I. The important diagnosis to exclude is an acute **compartment syndrome.** This occurs when the pressure within a compartment, in this case an osteofascial muscle compartment, exceeds the perfusion pressure. This leads to muscle and nerve ischaemia. If left untreated it can cause ischaemic muscle necrosis, limb contracture, renal failure or death.

II. There are **four** compartments in the leg. They are separated by the interosseous membrane and intermuscular septa. They are the:
- anterior compartment
- lateral compartment
- superficial posterior compartment
- deep posterior compartment.

III. The muscles in each compartment are given in Table 2.1.

Table 2.1

Compartment	Muscles
Anterior	Tibialis anterior Extensor digitorum longus Extensor hallucis longus Peroneus tertius
Lateral	Peroneus longus Peroneus brevis
Superficial posterior	Gastrocnemius Soleus Plantaris
Deep posterior	Popliteus Flexor digitorum longus Flexor hallucis longus Tibialis posterior

IV. The neurovascular structures which pass through each compartment are summarised in Table 2.2.

Table 2.2

Compartment	Artery	Nerves
Anterior	Anterior tibial artery	Deep fibular nerve
Lateral	Does not contain its own artery; its muscles are mainly supplied by branches of the fibular (peroneal) artery which runs in the posterior compartment of the leg	Superficial fibular nerve
Superficial posterior	Does not contain its own artery; its blood supply is derived from branches of the posterior tibial artery	Does not have its own nerve but is innervated by the tibial nerve
Deep posterior	Posterior tibial artery mainly	Tibial nerve

V. The gastrocnemius muscle contributes to a large tendon, the **calcaneal (Achilles) tendon** which, as its name suggests, inserts into the **calcaneus** (middle third). The other muscles which contribute to this tendon are the soleus and plantaris. Two bursae are present: one between the tendon and the upper part of the calcaneus and the other between the tendon and the deep fascia of the leg.

VI. See Image 2.14.

VII. Structure A is the **tibia**, and structure B is the **interosseous membrane**. The interosseous membrane separates the anterior and posterior compartments and provides an area of muscle attachment.

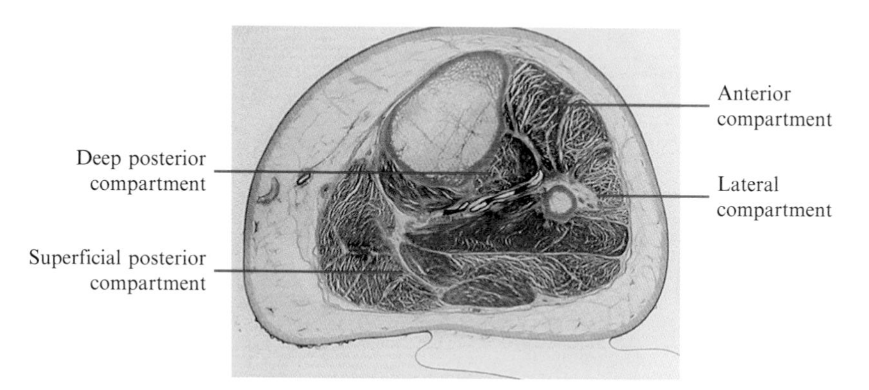

Image 2.14

VIII. Structures C and D are the **posterior tibial vein** and **artery**, with the tibial nerve also visible in this neurovascular bundle. The posterior tibial artery arises from the popliteal artery at the lower border of popliteus, passing under the fibrous arch in the origin of soleus to reach the deep posterior compartment of the leg.

IX. Muscle E is the **tibialis anterior**. It arises from the upper two-thirds of the lateral surface of the tibia and adjacent interosseous membrane and inserts into the medial cuneiform and the base of the first metatarsal. Tibialis anterior has two main actions: it **dorsiflexes** and **inverts** the foot.

X. Muscle F is the **gastrocnemius**, which has two heads. The medial head originates from the popliteal surface of the femur and a small pit on the back of the medial femoral condyle, and the lateral head originates from the lateral femoral condyle; the muscle bellies converge to insert into the calcaneus via the Achilles tendon. The two heads of gastrocnemius and the soleus are collectively known as the triceps surae. Their main action is to **plantarflex** the ankle. When walking or running, this action raises the heel propelling the body forwards. Gastrocnemius is also a **knee flexor**.

Question 11

I. See Image 2.15. Vertebral bodies strengthen the vertebral column and support the weight of the body. The bodies of lumbar vertebrae are large, wider transversely, forming a kidney shape, and deeper anteriorly. The anterior and posterior longitudinal ligaments help stabilise the spine. Intervertebral discs provide strong attachments between each vertebral body.

II. Spinous processes project posteriorly from the vertebral arch, and provide attachment for muscles of the back. The spinous processes of lumbar vertebrae are thick, short and protrude almost horizontally.

III. The pedicles make up part of the neural arch, connecting it to the vertebral body. They join the vertebral laminae posteriorly.

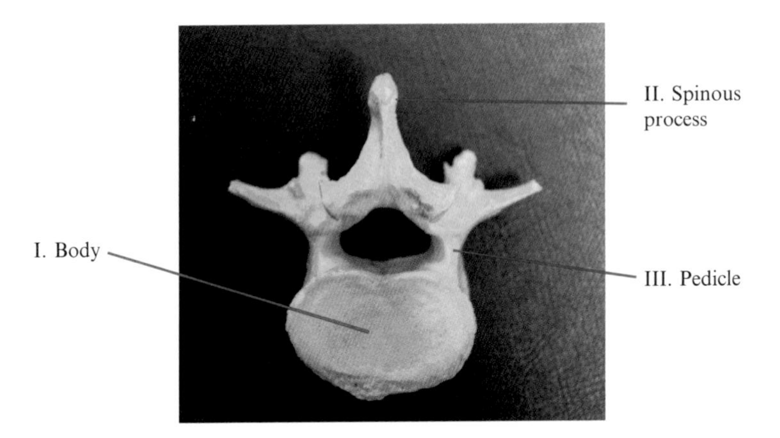

Image 2.15

IV. Typical cervical vertebrae (C3–6) have the following features:
- A **small, wide body**, which has a concave superior surface and a convex inferior surface.
- Transverse processes containing **transverse foramina** for passage of vertebral vessels (small or absent in C7). Transverse processes have anterior and posterior tubercles for muscle attachments.
- The superior articular facets **face obliquely** up and back, and the inferior articular facets are directed **down** and **forward**.
- The spinous process is **short** and **bifid** (C7 has the longest spinous process, hence the description vertebra prominens).

V. Intervertebral joints are **secondary cartilaginous joints**. Cartilaginous joints are characterised by bone ends covered by a layer of hyaline cartilage. In primary cartilaginous joints (synchondroses), such as epiphyses, there is only hyaline cartilage between the bone segments; whereas in secondary cartilaginous joints (symphyses) there is a layer of fibrocartilage between the hyaline cartilage covering the bone ends. All symphyses are found in the midline and include the manubriosternal joint and the pubic symphysis.

VI. See Image 2.16.

VII. The sagittal MRI scan shows a **prolapsed L4/5 intervertebral disc**. A prolapse is caused by herniation of the gelatinous nucleus pulposus through a weakened anulus fibrosus. The wedge shape of the disc and the eccentrically positioned nucleus pulposus directs most disc prolapses towards the posterior longitudinal ligament, which then deflects the herniation posterolaterally. A prolapse may occur as a result of degeneration or trauma.

VIII. A posterolateral L4/5 prolapse, the most common level of disc prolapse, usually causes pressure on the **L5 nerve root**, i.e. the spinal nerve emerging from the intervertebral foramen *one level below* that of the prolapse. Irritation of the L5 nerve root may therefore cause pain radiating down

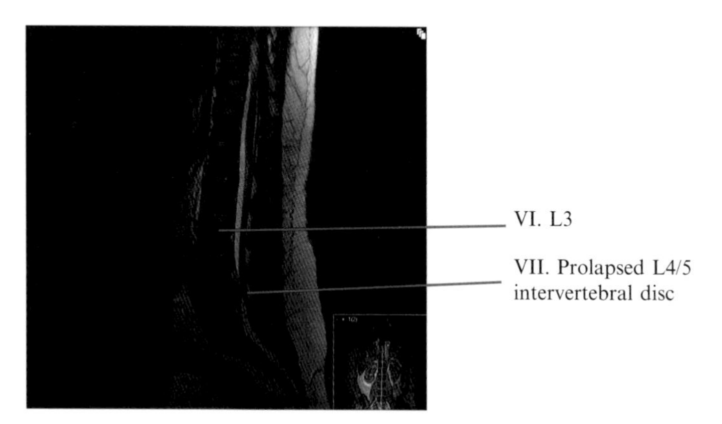

Image 2.16

the lower limb, weak ankle dorsiflexion and toe extension and numbness over the lateral leg, dorsum of the foot and great toe (the nerve root's distribution).

IX. The adult spinal cord ends **between L1 and L2**. It tapers into the cone-shaped conus medullaris, and the surrounding pia descends further as the fibrous filum terminale, which attaches to the coccyx.

X. The aim of a lumbar puncture is to remove cerebrospinal fluid from the subarachnoid space. The layers encountered during a lumbar puncture include:
   a. skin
   b. subcutaneous fat
   c. deep fascia
   d. supraspinous and interspinous ligaments (in midline)
   e. ligamentum flavum (to the side of the midline between the laminae)
   f. extradural space (fat and vessels)
   g. dura and arachnoid (no interval between the two).

ENDNOTES

1 Sir Charles Bell, 1774–1842, Scottish surgeon and anatomist, who also described Bell's facial palsy.
2 Friedrich Trendelenburg (1844–1924), German surgeon.
3 William Morrant Baker (1839–1896), British surgeon.

3

Thorax questions

Question 1

Scenario:
You are the surgical senior house officer on a cardiothoracic firm. A patient has a pneumothorax which requires decompression with a surgical chest drain.

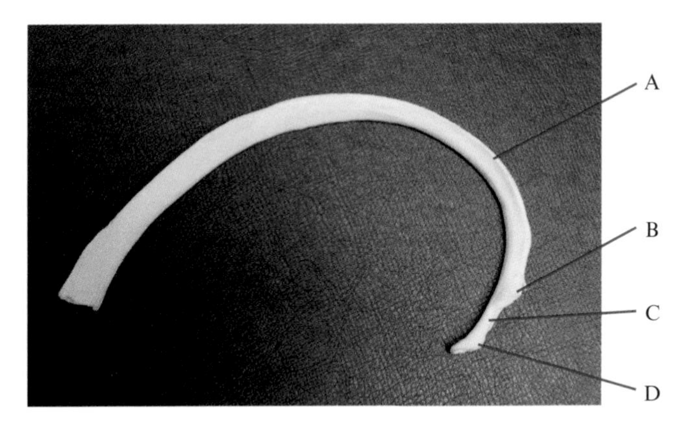

Image 3.1

With regards to Image 3.1:

I. What is structure A?
II. What is structure B, and with what does it articulate?
III. What is structure C?
IV. What is structure D, and what does it articulate?
V. In what order do the contents of the intercostal neurovascular bundle run?
VI. In which muscle plane do these structures run?
VII. In which direction do the fibres of the external intercostal muscles run?

VIII. Where is the 'safe zone' for insertion of a chest drain?
IX. What are the surface landmarks for the pleural reflections?
X. What are the surface landmarks for the oblique fissures?
XI. What are the surface landmarks for the horizontal fissure?

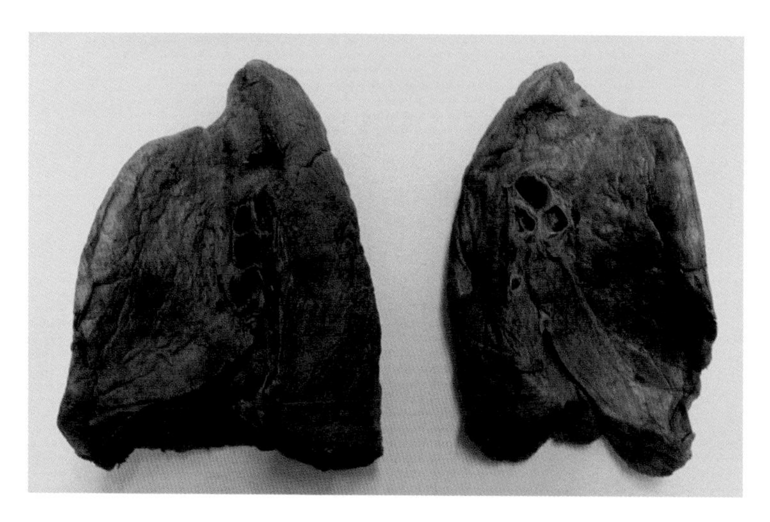

Image 3.2

XII. With regards to Image 3.2, label the following structures:
- The left and right pulmonary arteries.
- The left and right pulmonary veins.
- The left and right main bronchus or derivation.
- The left and right cardiac impressions.

XIII. How many lobes does each lung have?
XIV. What is a bronchopulmonary segment?
XV. Why would a lobe of a lung not infarct following a pulmonary embolism?

Question 2

Scenario:
A patient is brought into your A&E department having been stabbed in the chest. The single stab wound has penetrated the heart at the location indicated on Image 3.3.

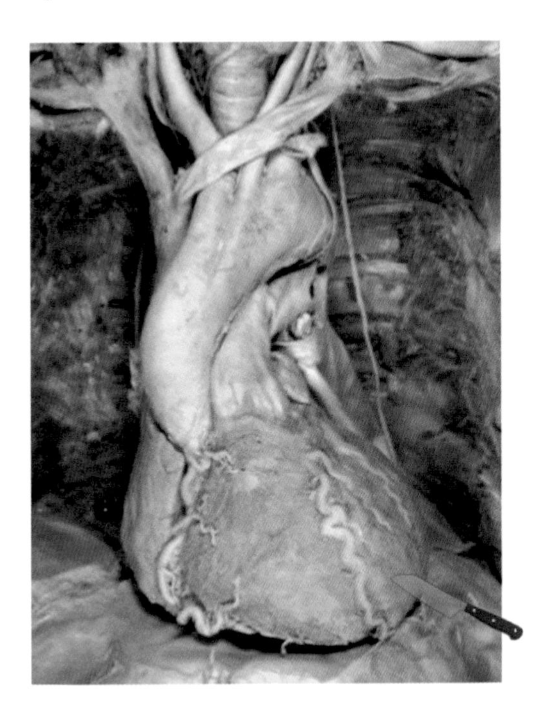

Image 3.3

I. What are the surface markings of the heart?

With regards to Image 3.3:

II. Where is the stab wound situated?

III. Point out the left auricle and the right ventricle.

IV. What valve separates the right ventricle from the pulmonary trunk?

V. How many cusps does this valve have?

VI. What coronary artery, running along the anterior interventricular border, could have been injured in this case?

VII. Identify the artery on Image 3.4, a coronary angiogram.

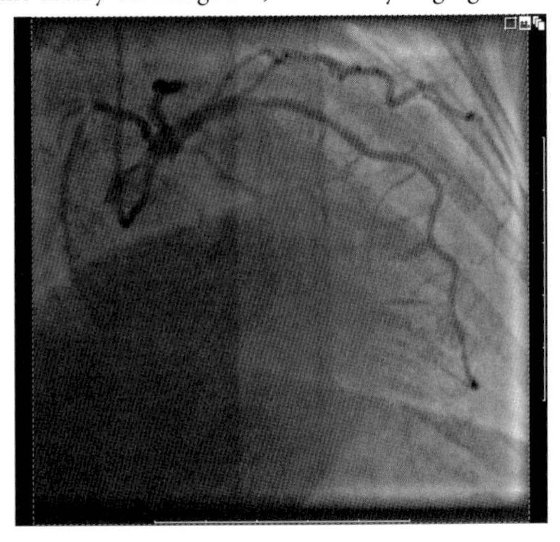

Image 3.4

VIII. Which coronary artery supplies the atrioventricular (AV) node in the majority of people?
IX. In which part of the mediastinum is the heart contained?
X. What are the boundaries of the mediastinum?
XI. What are the contents of the superior mediastinum?

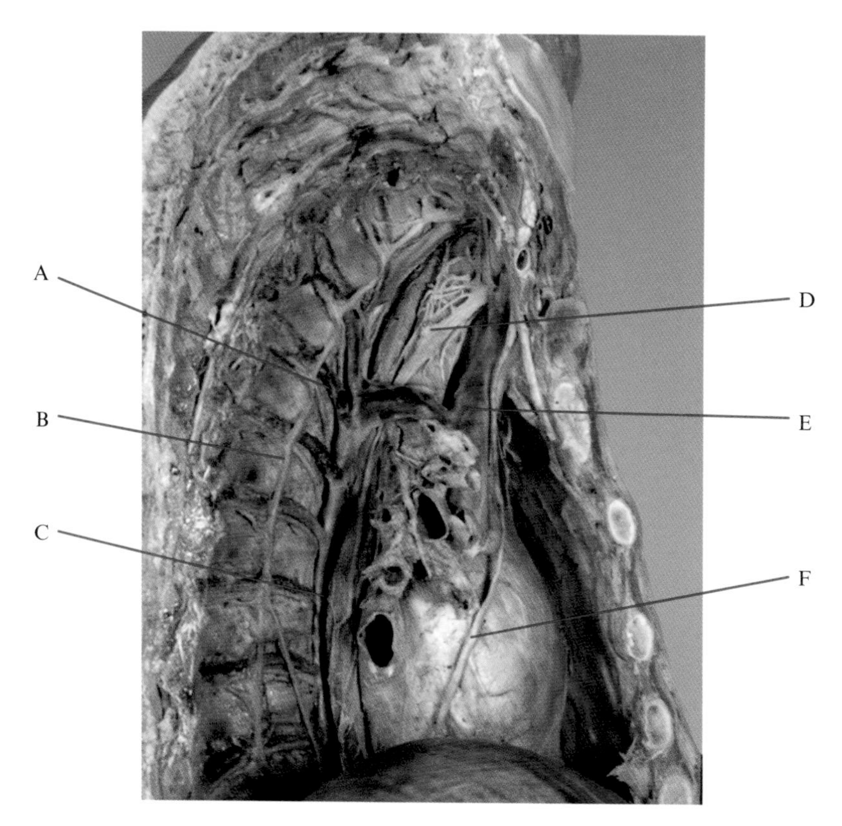

Image 3.5

With regards to Image 3.5:
XII. What is structure A?
XIII. What is structure B?
XIV. What is structure C?
XV. What is structure D?
XVI. What is structure E?
XVII. What is structure F, and what is its function?
XVIII. Label structures A–G on Image 3.6.

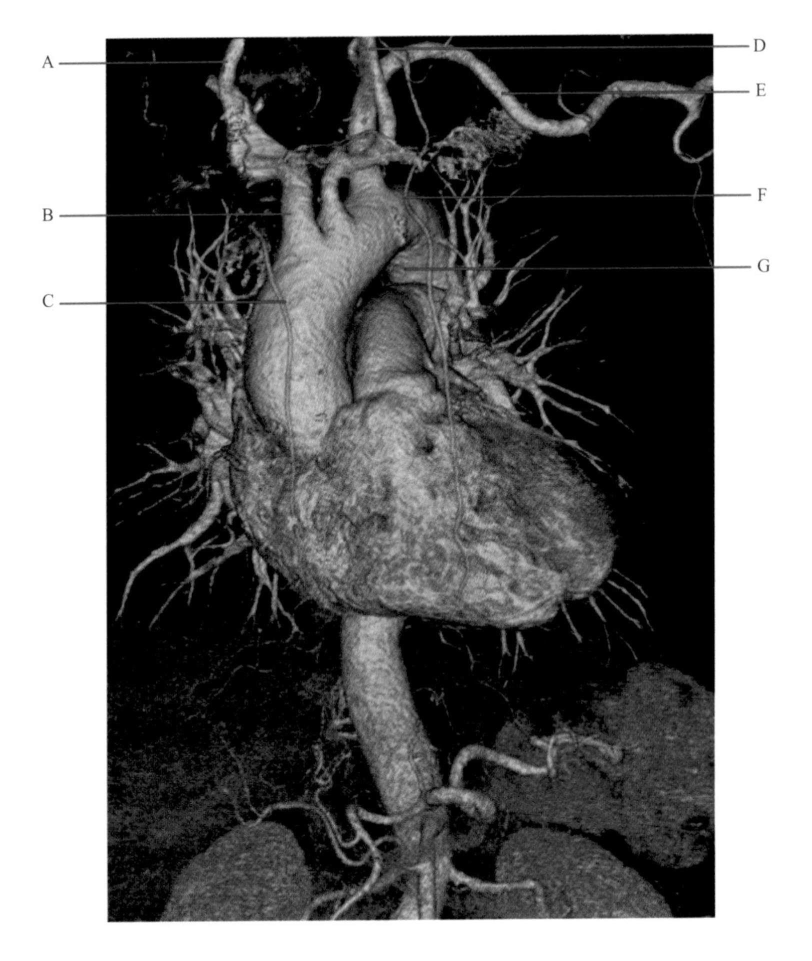

Image 3.6

Question 3

Scenario:
A patient presents to clinic complaining of weight loss and dysphagia. Following an endoscopy, a diagnosis of oesophageal cancer is made. It is affecting the distal third of his oesophagus.

With regards to Image 3.7:

I. Identify the left brachiocephalic vein.
II. Identify the arch of the aorta.

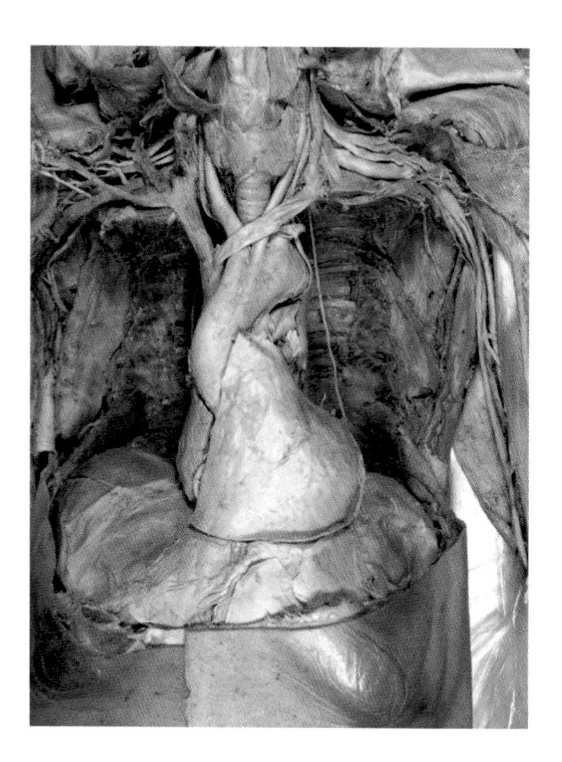

Image 3.7

III. Identify the right subclavian artery.
IV. Identify the left hemidiaphragm.
V. What movements does the diaphragm make during respiration?
VI. What are the diaphragm's attachments?
VII. What is the diaphragm's nerve supply?
VIII. How long is the oesophagus?
IX. In which part(s) of the mediastinum does the oesophagus run?
X. What are the relations of the oesophagus as it enters the mediastinum?
XI. At which points during its course does the oesophagus narrow?
XII. What layers make up the oesophageal wall?
XIII. Describe the blood supply to the oesophagus.
XIV. Describe the venous drainage of the oesophagus.
XV. What is the clinical significance of the venous drainage of the lower end of the oesophagus?
XVI. Does this phenomenon appear elsewhere?
XVII. At what level does the oesophagus pass through the diaphragm?
XVIII. At what level does the aorta pass through the diaphragm?
XIX. At what level does the inferior vena cava (IVC) pass through the diaphragm?

Question 4

Scenario:

You review a lady in an outpatient clinic who presents with a lump in her breast. A chaperone should be present in this scenario.

I. Examine this patient's axilla, demonstrating the various groups of axillary lymph nodes.
II. What is meant by the term 'level 3 node'?
III. What are the surface markings of the female breast?
IV. What is the blood supply to the breast?
V. What nerves are most at risk of injury in an axillary dissection?

4

Thorax answers

Question 1

I. Structure A is the **subcostal groove**. The subcostal groove lies on the inferior inner aspect of the rib. It conveys the neurovascular bundle.

II. Structure B is the **tubercle** of the rib, which is located at the junction of the neck and the shaft. It has a facet which articulates with the corresponding vertebral transverse process. An adjacent non-articular part of the facet gives attachment to the lateral costotransverse ligament.

III. Structure C is the **neck** of the rib, which connects the head and shaft. At its junction with the shaft, the articular facet of the tubercle protrudes posteriorly and externally.

IV. Structure D is the **head** of the rib. It has two facets which are separated by a transverse crest. These facets articulate with the bodies of their corresponding vertebra and with the vertebra above (the transverse crest is attached to the intervertebral disc).

V. The intercostal vein is most superior and the nerve the most inferior, with the artery in between. This can be remembered by the sequence **VAN**.

VI. These structures run between the **internal** and **innermost intercostal muscles**; i.e. between the middle and inner layers of muscles. This is similar to the vessels and nerves of the abdominal wall, which run between the internal oblique and transversus abdominis muscles.

VII. The external intercostal muscles run obliquely **downwards**, **forwards** and **medially** between two adjacent ribs. Their function is to elevate the ribs. In contrast, the internal intercostal fibres run at right angles to those of the external intercostals, and so run backwards, laterally and downwards. They act to depress ribs. The fibres of the innermost intercostal muscles cross more than one rib and may be absent in the upper thorax. All the intercostal muscles are innervated by the adjoining intercostal nerves.

VIII. Chest drains can be inserted within a ‘safe triangle’ bounded by the following landmarks:

- the anterior border of latissimus dorsi (which together with teres major forms the posterior axillary fold);
- the lateral border of pectoralis major (the anterior axillary fold);
- a horizontal line at the level of the nipple.

IX. The apex of the pleura lies 2.5 cm above the medial third of the clavicle. The parietal pleura can then be traced medially behind the sternoclavicular joint to meet the contralateral pleura at the sternal angle (of Louis[1]). On the right the pleura continues inferiorly towards the 6th costal cartilage before crossing the midclavicular line over the 8th rib and the midaxillary line over the 10th rib. On the left the pleura deviates laterally at the level of the 4th costal cartilage to overlie at the anterior end of the 6th rib. It then follows the same landmarks as the right pleura. From the midaxillary line, the inferior margin of the pleura passes to the 12th thoracic vertebra and passes over the diaphragm.

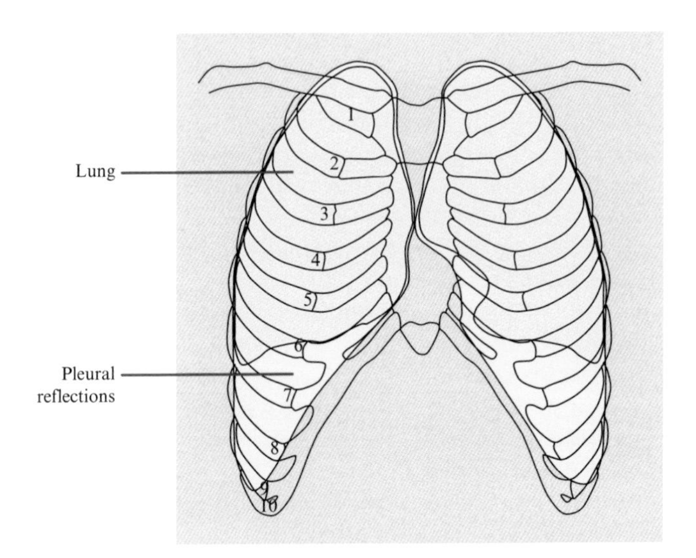

Image 4.1

X. The oblique fissure separates the upper and lower lobes of both left and right lungs. It can be marked approximately by a line from the posterior end of the third rib to the sixth costal cartilage in the midclavicular line. This crosses the midaxillary line over the fifth rib. This equates roughly to the medial border of the scapula when the arm is fully abducted.

XI. The horizontal fissure lies between the middle and upper lobes of the right lung. It can be approximately surface marked by a line joining the fourth costal cartilage and the oblique fissure where it crosses the fifth rib, at the midaxillary line.

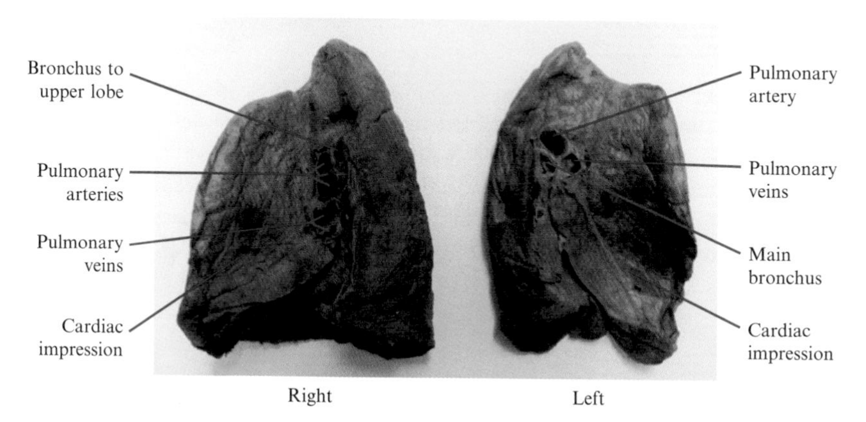

Image 4.2

XII. The root of the lung is shaped like a forward-facing inverted comma, the tail of which represents the pulmonary ligament and the body of which represents the hilum of the root of the lung. The bronchi lie posteriorly (the right lung root contains a separate superior and middle/inferior bronchus; whereas the left root contains one left main bronchus). The pulmonary artery lies superior (on the right the artery has already bifurcated whereas on the left it hasn't), and the pulmonary veins lie anteriorly and inferiorly, either side of the oblique fissure.

XIII. The right lung has three lobes:
- upper (three bronchopulmonary segments)
- middle (two bronchopulmonary segments)
- lower (five bronchopulmonary segments).

The left lung has two lobes:
- upper (five bronchopulmonary segments)
- lower (five bronchopulmonary segments).

XIV. Each lung lobe consists of a series of bronchopulmonary segments. A bronchopulmonary segment is a structurally separate, functionally independent unit of lung tissue with its own segmental bronchus and pulmonary artery branch. It is approximately pyramidal in shape with an apex pointing towards the apex of the lung.

XV. The bronchial arteries supply the bronchial tree, down to the respiratory bronchioles. The pulmonary circulation carries deoxygenated blood from the heart to the lungs for oxygenation, and back to the heart. A pulmonary embolus occludes pulmonary arterial branches but does not interrupt the bronchial circulation, which continues to supply much of the pulmonary parenchyma and therefore protects against major regions of infarction.

Question 2

I. The heart can be mapped by joining four points, in a trapezoid shape. The superior border is formed by a line joining the left second costal cartilage and the right third costal cartilage, 1 cm lateral to the respective sternal edges. The right border then descends in a curved line to a point 1–2 cm lateral to the right sternal edge, to the level of the sixth costal cartilage. The inferior border joins this point to the apex of the heart, at the fifth intercostal space, midclavicular line. The lateral border then curves, slightly convex laterally, towards the second intercostal space.

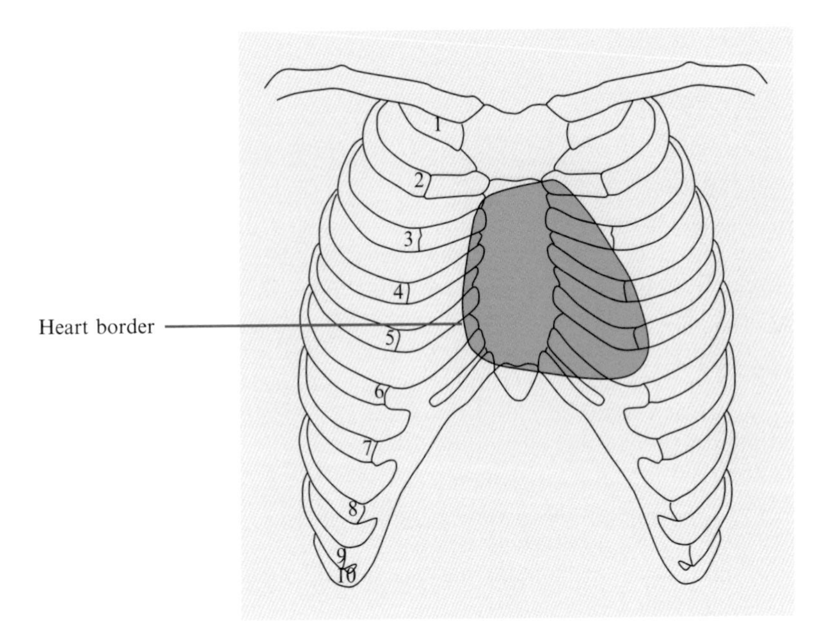

Image 4.3

II. The stab wound is located in the **left ventricle**.

III. The left auricle (or left atrial appendage) is a muscular pouch attached to the left atrium. It functions as a reservoir of the left atrium. Approximately 90% of clots which develop in atrial fibrillation arise from the left auricle. The pulmonary trunk transmits deoxygenated blood from the right ventricle of the heart to the lungs. It is approximately 5 cm long and 3 cm wide, and is the most anterior of the great vessels.

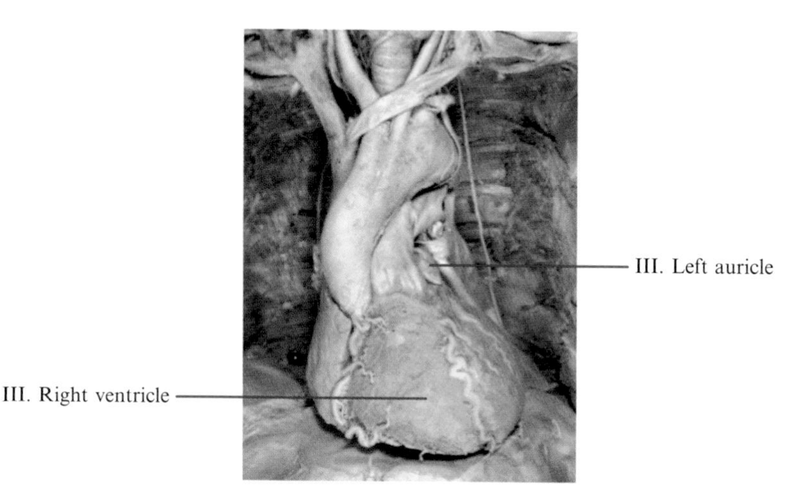

Image 4.4

IV. The **pulmonary valve** lies approximately at the level of the left third costal cartilage and is the semilunar valve at the outflow from the right ventricle.

V. The pulmonary valve has **three cusps** – a right, left and an anterior cusp. Like the aortic valve, it is a passive valve, opening in systole and closing in diastole.

VI. The **left anterior descending** (**LAD**) artery runs in the anterior interventricular groove of the heart towards the apex. It lies just medial to the knife wound.

VII. Image 4.5 demonstrates the LAD artery. The LAD artery is a branch of the left main stem (LMS), the other branch being the circumflex artery. The left main stem arises from the ostium of the left coronary sinus (of Valsalva[2]) and travels between the pulmonary trunk and left auricular appendage, before reaching the atrioventricular groove, where it usually divides into two main branches. The left anterior descending artery is one of these major branches and it runs in the anterior interventricular groove. Different angiographic views will depict the arteries of the left system in different positions. Remember that the LAD artery will travel to the apex of the heart (and is thus the longest vessel) and has septal branches coming off it at right angles. The circumflex is shorter and is always positioned closest to the spine.

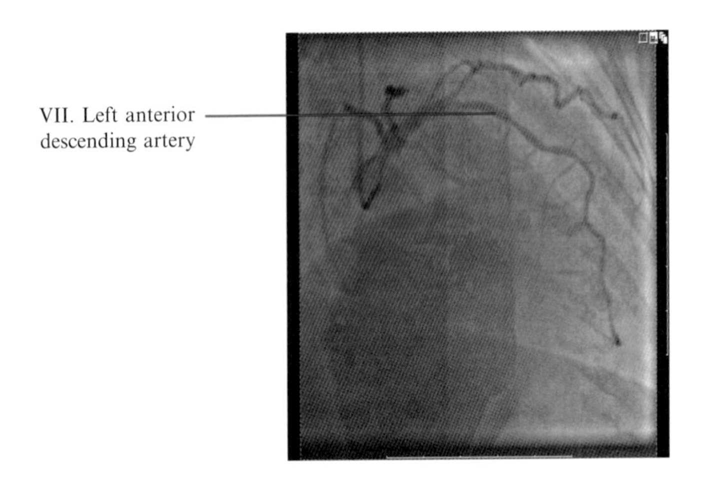

Image 4.5

VIII. The **right coronary artery** supplies the AV node in approximately 80% of patients and the sinoatrial (SA) node in approximately 60% of patients.

IX. The heart is contained in the **middle mediastinum** along with the following structures:
- pericardial sac (which acts as a boundary)
- the arch of the azygos vein
- the roots of the great vessels
- the bifurcation of the trachea and both main bronchi
- lymph nodes and the phrenic nerves.

X. The mediastinum is the region between the lungs. It is bounded by the following structures:
- the superior thoracic aperture (often called the thoracic inlet)
- the diaphragm (inferiorly)
- the sternum (anteriorly)
- the thoracic vertebrae (posteriorly).

It can be subdivided into the superior and inferior mediastinum by a horizontal line through the sternal angle, equating to the inferior portion of the fourth thoracic vertebrae; this line is sometimes referred to as the transverse thoracic plane. The inferior mediastinum is subdivided further by the heart into the anterior, middle and posterior divisions.

XI. The contents of the superior mediastinum include the following:
- arch of the aorta and its branches
- superior vena cava (upper part)
- brachiocephalic veins
- trachea
- oesophagus
- thymus

- vagus nerves and phrenic nerves
- left recurrent laryngeal nerve
- internal thoracic vessels
- thoracic duct and tracheobronchial lymph nodes.

XII. **Posterior intercostal veins and arteries**. There are 11 pairs of posterior intercostal vessels which run along the subcostal grooves, the vein superior to the artery. The vein also drains blood from the muscles of the back.

XIII. **Sympathetic trunk**. Each sympathetic trunk is a ganglionated nerve cord which travels from just below the base of the skull to the coccyx. Anterior to the coccyx the two trunks meet to form a single, median, terminal ganglion (ganglion impar). In the thorax the sympathetic trunks lie mostly anterior to the heads of the ribs.

XIV. **Azygos vein**. The azygos system drains blood from the posterior walls of the thorax and abdomen into the superior vena cava (SVC). The azygos vein is formed at the level of T12 by the union of the ascending lumbar veins and the right subcostal veins. It receives the hemiazygos vein and accessory hemiazygos vein in its course.

XV. **Vagus nerve**. The vagus nerve is the 10th cranial nerve (CN X). The course of the left and right nerves differs slightly in the thorax. The right nerve passes posterior to the right brachiocephalic vein, SVC and right lung root. The left vagus nerve enters the thorax between the left common carotid and left subclavian arteries, behind the left brachiocephalic vein. It gives off the left recurrent laryngeal nerve at the inferior border of the arch of the aorta and then travels posterior to the root of the left lung.

XVI. The **superior vena cava**. This picture demonstrates the azygos vein draining into the SVC, which itself empties into the right atrium.

XVII. The **phrenic nerves** provide the sole motor supply to the diaphragm. Each nerve enters the mediastinum anterior to the subclavian artery. The left nerve can be found behind, and the right nerve to the left of, the origin of the brachiocephalic vein. The phrenic nerves can easily be distinguished from the vagus nerves, as they travel anterior to the root of the lung; whereas the vagus nerves travel posterior to it.

XVIII. This is an enhanced CT aortogram. The aorta arches at the level of the sternal angle posterosuperiorly and towards the left. This can make the distinction between the left common carotid and left subclavian artery difficult to visualise when looking at the vessels square on. The labelled structures are:

A. Right common carotid artery
B. Brachiocephalic trunk
C. Aortic arch
D. Left common carotid artery
E. Left subclavian artery
F. Left internal thoracic artery
G. Descending aorta.

Question 3

I. See Image 4.6.
II. See Image 4.6.
III. See Image 4.6.
IV. See Image 4.6.

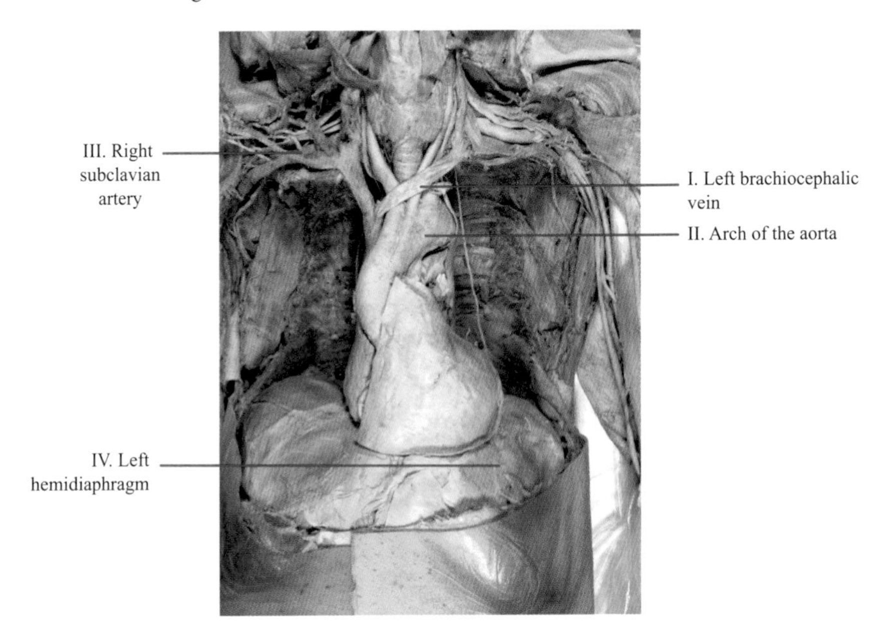

Image 4.6

V. The diaphragm is a dome-shaped muscular structure which separates the thorax from the abdomen. It consists of a trifoliate aponeurotic central tendon and a peripheral muscular section. It has a major role to play in respiration. During inspiration the central portion of the diaphragm descends, and in expiration it ascends as high as the fifth rib on the right and fifth intercostal space on the left.

VI. The muscular part of the diaphragm is grouped according to the origin of its muscle fibres:

- **Vertebral part** – the vertebral part forms the arcuate ligaments and the crura of the diaphragm. The fibres forming the crura arise from the bodies of the lumbar vertebrae (the right crus from L1–3 and the left crus from L1–2). The medial borders of the crura then form the median arcuate ligament. The medial arcuate ligament is formed by the thickening of the fascia overlying psoas major, and the lateral arcuate ligament by the fascia overlying quadratus lumborum.
- **Costal part** – the inner aspects of the inferior six ribs give rise to the costal part of the diaphragm.

- **Sternal part** – two small slips originate from the deep surface of the xiphisternum.

VII. The diaphragm is innervated by the **phrenic nerve**. Its nerve root values are C3,4,5, the most significant contribution originating from C4.

VIII. The oesophagus is approximately **25 cm long**, running from the lower border of the cricoid cartilage, at the level of C6, to the cardiac orifice of the stomach, at the level of T11.

IX. The oesophagus runs in the **superior** and **posterior** parts of the mediastinum.

X. The oesophagus enters the mediastinum between the trachea and the vertebral column, initially slightly to the left. It then is pushed towards the midline by the aortic arch, which therefore lies to its left. The thoracic duct also lies to the left of the oesophagus at this level, deep to the aortic arch.

XI. The oesophagus has four areas of constriction. They are:
a. at its beginning – around 15 cm from the incisors;
b. where the aortic arch crosses – around 22 cm from the incisors;
c. where the left main bronchus crosses – around 27 cm from the incisors;
d. as it passes through the diaphragm – around 38–40 cm from the incisors.
These areas are clinically important as they may be the areas in which a foreign body may impact. The position of the beginning of the oesophagus and the level at which it passes through the diaphragm are reasonably reliable measures; however, the two narrowings in between are quite variable.

XII. The oesophageal wall is made of the following layers (from the lumen, outwards):
a. **Mucosa**. This consists of the following layers:
  1. **Epithelium** – this is non-keratinised, stratified squamous epithelium which ends abruptly, giving rise to the columnar epithelium of the stomach. This layer provides a good protection against mechanical injury as it is thick and lined with mucous. Squamous cells are, however sensitive to substances such as alcohol and tobacco and certain dietary factors, predisposing the oesophagus to squamous cell carcinomas. Furthermore, squamous cells are sensitive to the acidic and protease-rich stomach secretions which may cause intestinal metaplasia of the squamous cells to a columnar epithelial mucosa. This intestinal metaplasia leads to Barrett's oesophagus, which is a precursor to adenocarcinoma. The increase in gastro-oesophageal reflux disease in Western society has led to an increase in the proportion of adenocarcinomas in comparison to squamous cell carcinomas.
  2. **Lamina propria** – containing mucosa-associated lymphoid tissue.
  3. **Muscularis mucosa** – this layer contains longitudinal smooth muscle sheets which are thinner in the proximal oesophagus, i.e. near the pharynx, and become thicker distally, closer to the gastro-oesophageal junction.

b. **Submucosa** – a layer which loosely connects the mucosa and muscularis externa. It contains mucous glands, vessels and nerves.

c. **Muscularis externa** – this layer contains an inner circular layer and an outer longitudinal layer, similar in arrangement to the intestine.

XIII. There are three main vascular territories of the oesophagus. They are:
a. cervical oesophagus – supplied by the **inferior thyroid artery**;
b. thoracic oesophagus – supplied by branches of the **thoracic aorta**;
c. abdominal oesophagus – supplied via the **left gastric artery**.

XIV. As with the arterial supply, the venous drainage is split into three main territories. They are:
a. cervical oesophagus – **inferior thyroid veins**;
b. thoracic oesophagus – **azygos vein**;
c. abdominal oesophagus – **azygos vein** and **left gastric veins**.

XV. The lower end of the oesophagus drains into both the systemic circulation (azygos vein) and the portal circulation (left gastric vein), and in doing so forms a portosystemic anastomosis. During periods of portal hypertension, collateral veins distend and form large portosystemic collaterals, or oesophageal varices. These may rupture causing an upper gastrointestinal bleed.

XVI. Other sites of portosystemic anastomosis, which may become pathological, include the following:
- **Rectum** – between superior rectal vein (drains to inferior mesenteric vein and then to the portal vein) and middle/inferior rectal veins (drain to internal iliac veins and therefore the systemic circulation). These can be seen along the rectal wall but only rarely bleed.
- **Periumbilical** – paraumbilical tributaries of the portal vein (portal) and branches of superior and inferior epigastric veins (systemic). These may lead to the formation of a caput medusa.
- **Retroperitoneal** – right, middle and left colic veins (portal), and renal, suprarenal, paravertebral and gonadal veins (systemic).

XVII. The oesophagus passes through the diaphragm at the level of the **T10**, along with:
- anterior and posterior vagal trunks
- oesophageal branches of the left gastric vessels
- lymphatic vessels.

The oesophageal aperture is bounded by muscle fibres from the right crus of the diaphragm.

XVIII. Strictly speaking, the aorta passes behind and not through the diaphragm at the level of **T12**. The so-called aortic opening is bounded posteriorly by the inferior portion of the T12 vertebra and the intervertebral disc, laterally by the crura of the diaphragm and anteriorly by the median arcuate ligament. Other structures passing through the aortic hiatus include:
- azygos and hemiazygos veins (this is variable)
- thoracic duct.

XIX. The IVC passes through the vena caval opening, the highest of the diaphragmatic apertures, at the level of the **T8/9** intervertebral disc. It is contained within the central tendon of the diaphragm, to the right of the median plane, where the tendons of the right and middle leaves meet. The IVC is adherent to the diaphragm and, during inspiration, when the

diaphragm contracts, the IVC expands, reducing caval pressure. This aids venous return. Along with the IVC, the vena caval hiatus transmits:
- terminal branches of the right phrenic nerve
- lymphatics.

Question 4

I. The axilla receives more than 75% of the lymphatic drainage of the breast, the rest draining mainly to the internal thoracic nodes. There are approximately 20–40 nodes which are not completely distinct from each other. These can be grouped into the following:
- **Anterior (pectoral) group** – along the inferolateral border of pectoralis minor, deep to pectoralis major.
- **Posterior (subscapular) group** – along the subscapular vessels.
- **Lateral group** – along the axillary vein.
- **Central group** – within the axillary fat behind pectoralis minor. These nodes receive lymphatics from the anterior, posterior and lateral groups, as well as directly from the breast itself.
- **Apical group** – at the apex of the axilla, above pectoralis minor and behind the clavicle. Efferents from the aforementioned groups drain into the apical group, along with lymphatics directly from the breast.

II. Clinically, nodes are referred to as being at one of three levels. These are as follows:
level 1 – below/inferior to pectoralis minor
level 2 – behind pectoralis minor
level 3 – between the upper border of pectoralis minor and the lower border of the clavicle.

III. The surface markings of the female breast are such that it overlies a region over the second to sixth ribs, over the fascia of the pectoralis major and serratus anterior muscles. Inferiorly the breast extends to overlie the external oblique aponeurosis. The axillary tail may extend into the axilla.

IV. The breast is supplied by the following arteries:
- The **axillary artery**, through its branches: superior thoracic, lateral thoracic, acromiothoracic (pectoral branch) and subscapular arteries.
- **Internal thoracic artery**.
- **Anterior intercostal arteries** (second to fourth).

V. In axillary dissections the following nerves are most at risk of injury:
- **long thoracic nerve** (supplying serratus anterior);
- **thoracodorsal nerve** (supplying latissimus dorsi);
- **medial** and **lateral pectoral nerves** (supply the pectoralis muscles);
- **intercostobrachial nerves** (cutaneous function).

The brachial plexus should be reasonably safe since axillary dissection is usually performed up to the level of the axillary vein.

ENDNOTES

1 Antoine Louis (1723–1792), French surgeon and physiologist.
2 Antonio Maria Valsalva (1666–1723), Italian anatomist.

5

Abdomen and pelvis questions

Question 1

Scenario:

A 21-year-old male presents with rebound tenderness in his right iliac fossa following a day of generalised abdominal discomfort. A diagnosis of acute appendicitis is made, and the patient is scheduled for an emergency open appendicectomy.

I. What are the surface markings for the base of a normally positioned appendix?
II. What layers would you dissect through when approaching an appendix through a muscle-splitting incision?
III. Why does the pain from appendicitis typically begin as a central abdominal pain but subsequently localise to the right iliac fossa?
IV. In what positions may the tip of the appendix lie?
V. With regards to closing a midline laparotomy incision, what does Jenkins' rule state?
VI. What are the attachments of the external oblique muscle?
VII. In which direction do the fibres of the external oblique muscle run?
VIII. What nerves innervate the external oblique muscle?

With regards to Image 5.1:

IX. Identify the external oblique muscle in the dissection.
X. In which direction do the fibres of the internal oblique muscle run?
XI. What are the attachments of the internal oblique muscle?
XII. What is the nerve supply to the internal oblique muscle?
XIII. What are the functions of the internal and external oblique muscles?
XIV. What is the conjoint tendon and where does it attach?
XV. What makes up the anterior rectus sheath:
   (a) above the umbilicus;
   (b) just above the pubis?

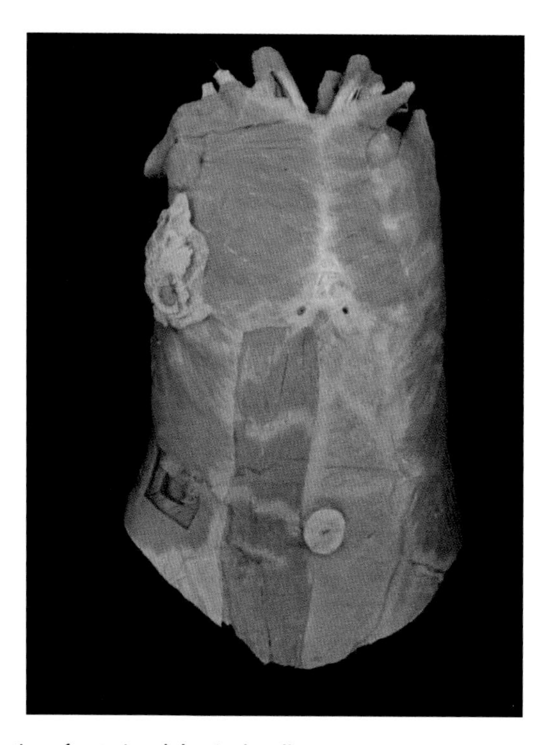

Image 5.1 Dissection of anterior abdominal wall

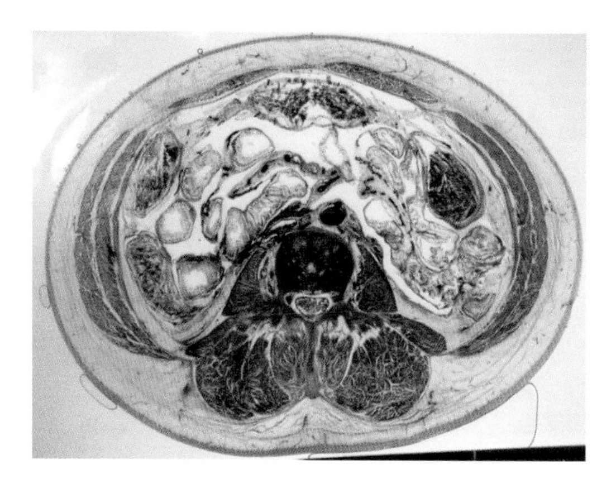

Image 5.2 Plastinated axial abdominal slice

With regards to Image 5.2:

XVI. In this sectional slice, identify the anterior rectus sheath.
XVII. Is this slice from above or below the arcuate line?
XVIII. Identify the muscle plane in which the abdominal wall nerves and vessels lie.
XIX. Identify the aorta.

XX. Identify the inferior vena cava (IVC).

In a patient with an inguinal hernia:

XXI. Where is the deep inguinal ring?
XXII. What are the boundaries of the inguinal canal?
XXIII. What are the boundaries of Hesselbach's inguinal triangle?
XXIV. What is the significance of this triangle in a patient with an inguinal hernia?

Question 2

Scenario:
A patient is admitted with colicky abdominal pain, vomiting and abdominal distension. They have previously had a laparotomy, the indication for which is unknown.

I. What is the most likely diagnosis?
II. What are the anatomical differences between the small and large bowel?
III. If the patient is taken to theatre for a laparotomy, how may the surgeon distinguish between the jejunum and the ileum?
IV. How is the duodenojejunal flexure identified intraoperatively?
V. Describe the parts of the duodenum.
VI. Is any section of the duodenum covered by a mesentery? Explain your answer.
VII. In a penetrating posterior duodenal ulcer, which vessel is at risk of causing a major haemorrhage?

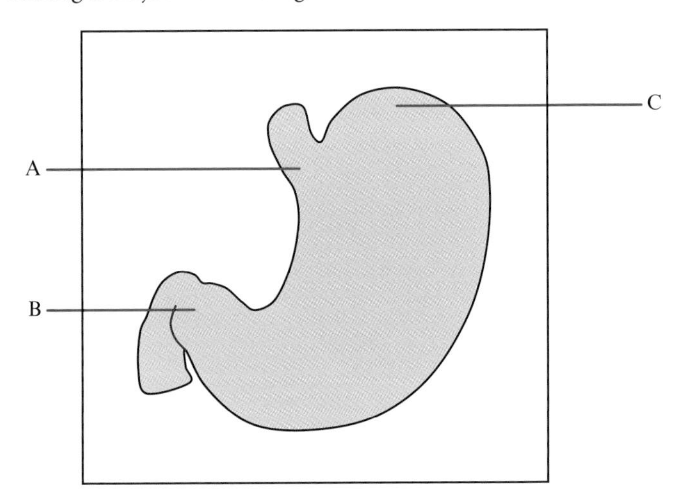

Image 5.3

With regards to Image 5.3:

VIII. What does A represent?
IX. What does B represent?
X. What does C represent?

XI. What arteries supply the lesser curvature of the stomach?
XII. What arteries supply the pancreas?
XIII. Is the pancreas intraperitoneal or retroperitoneal?
XIV. List the functions of the pancreas.

Question 3

Scenario:
You are examining a patient in whom you find an enlarged liver.

I. How many anatomical lobes does the liver have? What separates the lobes?
II. How is the liver functionally divided into left and right halves, and how is this plane represented on the surface of the liver?
III. How many functional segments does the liver have?
IV. Why is this relevant to a hepatobiliary surgeon?
V. Describe the blood supply to the liver.
VI. In what structure do these vessels travel to reach the liver?
VII. Following haemorrhage from the liver what manoeuvre can be performed intraoperatively to control bleeding?
VIII. How many hepatic veins are there?

With regards to Image 5.4:

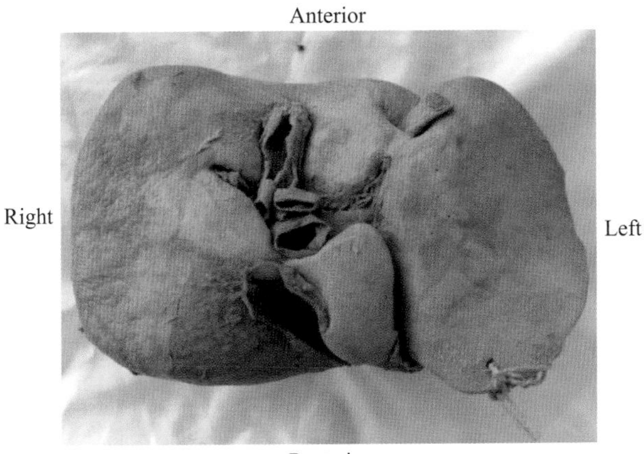

Image 5.4 **Visceral surface of liver**

IX. Identify the area of the liver related to the stomach.
X. Identify the area of attachment of the lesser omentum.
XI. Identify the caudate lobe.
XII. Identify the inferior vena cava (IVC).
XIII. Identify the area of the liver related to the kidney.
XIV. Identify the quadrate lobe.
XV. Identify the gallbladder.
XVI. What artery supplies the gallbladder?

Question 4

Scenario:
A 60-year-old hypertensive male presents in shock with abdominal pain radiating to his back. The axial CT shown in Image 5.5 is obtained.

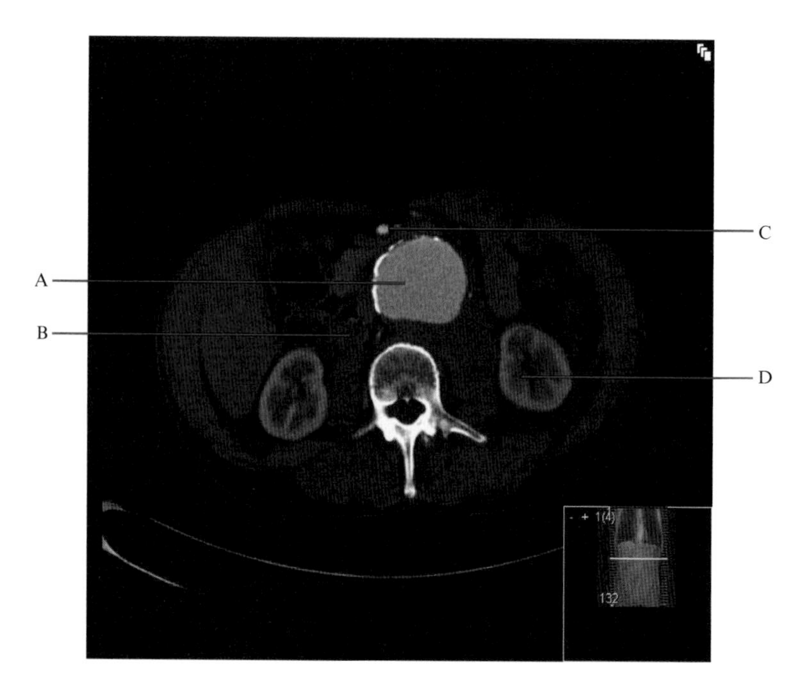

Image 5.5

With regards to Image 5.5:

I. What is structure A?
II. What is structure B?
III. What is structure C?
IV. What is structure D?

With regards to Image 5.6:

V. Identify the abdominal aorta.
VI. Identify the right common iliac artery.
VII. At what vertebral level does the aorta bifurcate?
VIII. What surface landmark(s) can be used to identify the aortic bifurcation?
IX. Identify the left renal vein.
X. At what vertebral level do the renal arteries originate?
XI. What are the relations of the renal arteries?
XII. What part of the pancreas is an anterior relation of the aorta?

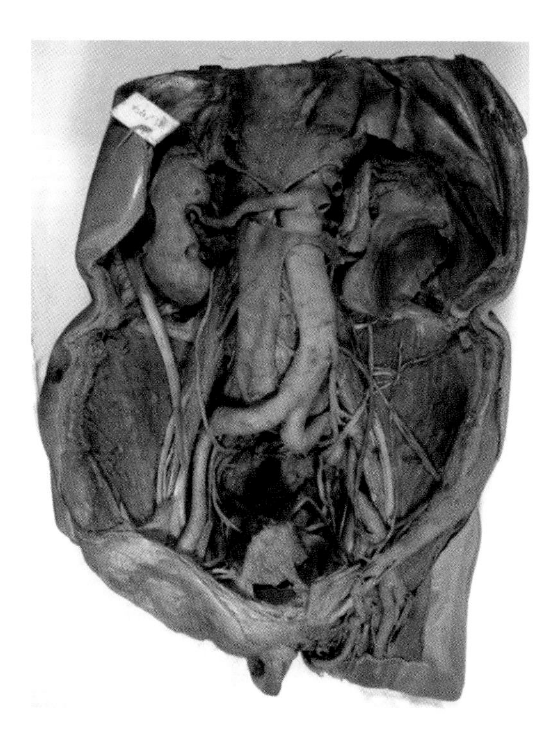

Image 5.6

XIII. Name the anterior unpaired branches of the aorta.
XIV. Identify these anterior unpaired branches in the dissection.
XV. The patient subsequently underwent an endovascular repair of his aortic aneurysm (EVAR). The graft excluded his inferior mesenteric artery (IMA) but he developed no signs of bowel ischaemia. What maintains the arterial supply to the hindgut when the IMA is occluded?
XVI. Identify the inferior vena cava.
XVII. At what vertebral level does the IVC begin?
XVIII. What are the main tributaries of the IVC?

Question 5

Scenario:
A 15-year-old male presents complaining of pain in his abdomen and left shoulder after a sporting injury. He is pale and clammy, with a pulse rate of 130 bpm and a blood pressure of 85/55 mmHg. A FAST (focused assessment with sonography for trauma) scan shows free fluid in the abdomen.

I. How would you manage this patient in the acute setting?
II. Why would a ruptured spleen cause shoulder tip pain?
III. What is the arterial supply to the spleen?

IV. Why is the spleen susceptible to rupture?
V. What are the surface landmarks of the spleen?
VI. What are the inferomedial relations of the spleen?

Question 6

Scenario:
A 40-year-old female presents to A&E with severe abdominal pain which radiates from her right flank to her groin. She has microscopic haematuria.

I. What is the most likely diagnosis?
II. Where in the ureter is a calculus most likely to become impacted?

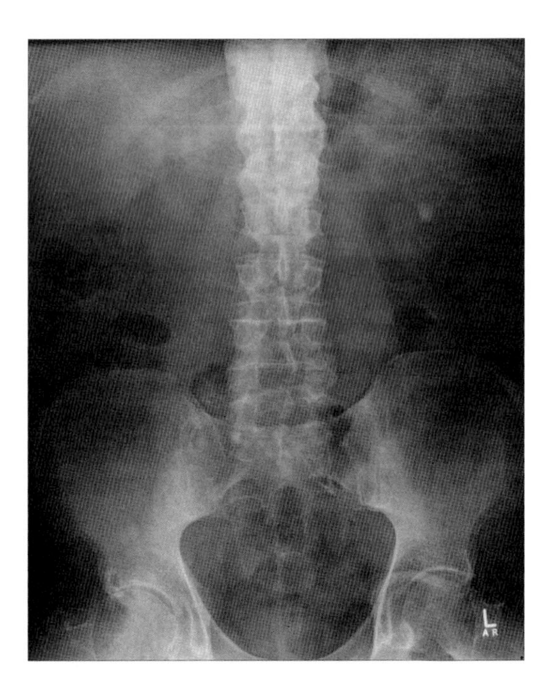

Image 5.7

III. On the radiograph in Image 5.7, identify the radiologic landmarks of a ureter as it descends from the kidney to the bladder.
IV. What is the arterial supply to the ureter?
V. Into which part of the bladder do the ureters enter?
VI. What type of epithelium lines the bladder?
VII. What are the posterior relations of the bladder in men?
VIII. What are the posterior relations of the bladder in women?
IX. Describe the parts of the male urethra.
X. Where does the epithelial lining change along the course of the male urethra?

6

Abdomen and pelvis answers

Question 1

I. The base of a normal appendix is stated to lie at **McBurney's point**,[1] which is sited two-thirds of the way along a line from the umbilicus to the anterior superior iliac spine. However, studies of normal appendices have shown that this surface marking is not particularly reliable.

II. The layers encountered in reaching the appendix through a right iliac fossa muscle-splitting incision are:
   a. skin
   b. subcutaneous fat (including Scarpa's fascia)
   c. external oblique aponeurosis (which should be cut in the line of its fibres)
   d. internal oblique muscle
   e. transversus abdominus muscle
   f. transversalis fascia
   g. extraperitoneal fat
   h. parietal peritoneum.

III. Colicky central abdominal pain is a common early symptom of acute appendicitis. This is referred pain due to the **visceral innervation** of the appendix, which is a midgut structure. The midgut extends from the second part of the duodenum to the distal transverse colon. As the appendiceal inflammation progresses, the overlying **parietal peritoneum** becomes inflamed. Since this is innervated by somatic nerves, localised pain develops in the right iliac fossa; i.e. the pain is experienced as shifting from the periumbilical region to the right iliac fossa.

IV. The vermiform appendix is a narrow tube which arises from the postero-medial aspect of the caecum, just inferior to the ileocaecal junction. The length of the appendix varies, and can be anything from 1 cm to more than 20 cm. The position of the tip of the appendix also varies, and precise figures for each position are notoriously variable between different series. However, classifications usually mention the following:

a. **retrocaecal** (behind the caecum) or **retrocolic** (behind the inferior ascending colon);
b. **subcaecal** (below the caecum) or **pelvic** (extending beyond the pelvic brim);
c. **retro-ileal** (behind the ileum) and **pre-ileal** (in front of the ileum).

Retrocaecal and pelvic are the two most common positions for the tip of the appendix in acute appendicitis. The position of the appendix may affect the clinical presentation of acute appendicitis. For example, a retrocaecal appendicitis may be shielded from the peritoneum by a caecum distended with bowel gas, causing little in the way of muscular rigidity or tenderness on deep palpation. A retrocaecal appendicitis may be in contact with the right psoas muscle and therefore cause pain on extension of the hip (psoas stretch sign). A pelvic appendicitis may inflame the rectum, causing diarrhoea, or the bladder causing dysuria (and a sterile pyuria). A retro-ileal appendicitis may inflame the distal ileum and also cause diarrhoea.

V. Jenkins' rule[2] states that, when closing a midline laparotomy incision, the length of suture should be four times the length of the wound, and each bite of the rectus sheath should contain a minimum of 1 cm of tissue and be at 1 cm intervals. Jenkins demonstrated that the length of an incision can increase postoperatively by up to 30%. If the bites and length of the suture are inadequate, the suture may cut through the fascia, causing a wound dehiscence.

VI. The attachments of the external oblique muscle are as follows:
- Origin – the external surfaces of the lower eight ribs. Its fibres interdigitate with those of serratus anterior above and latissimus dorsi below.
- Insertion – xiphisternum, linea alba, pubic tubercle, anterior half of the iliac crest. The external oblique has a free muscular posterior border.
- The inguinal ligament is formed by the guttered aponeurotic margin of the external oblique muscle between the anterior superior iliac spine and the pubic tubercle.

VII. The fibres of the external oblique muscle run in an **inferomedial direction**, between the attachments described above.

VIII. The **lower five intercostal nerves** and the **subcostal nerves** innervate the external oblique muscles (T7–12).

IX. See Image 6.1.

X. The internal oblique muscle fibres run at **right angles** to the external oblique fibres, passing upwards and medially.

XI. The attachments of the internal oblique muscle are as follows:
- Origin – lateral two-thirds of the inguinal ligament, anterior two-thirds of the iliac crest and thoracolumbar fascia.
- Insertion – inferior borders of the lower four ribs and their cartilages, the linea alba and, by way of the conjoint tendon, to the pubic crest and pectineal line.

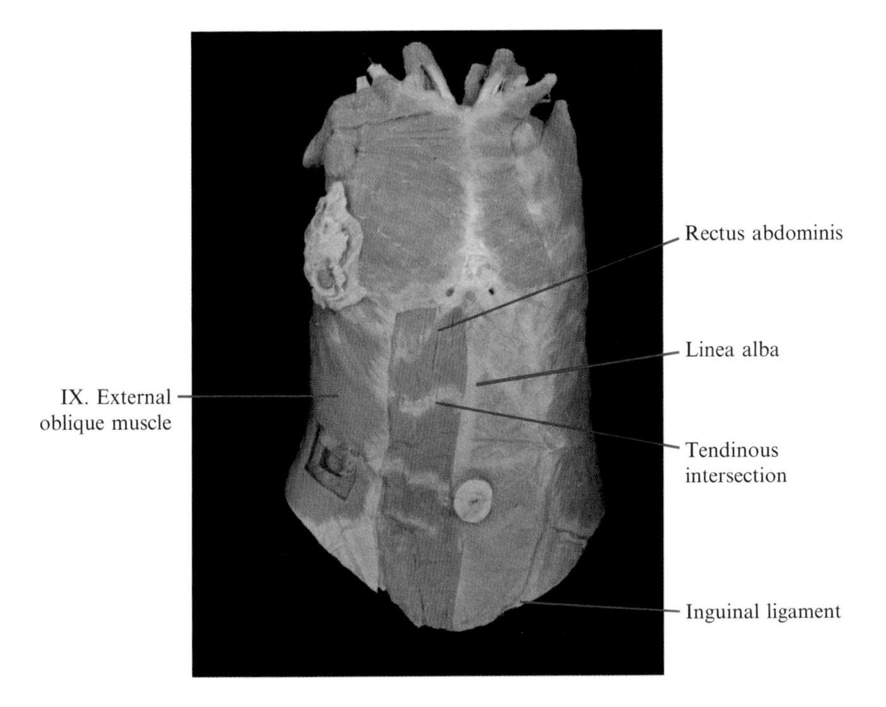

Image 6.1

XII. Both the internal oblique muscle and the transversus abdominis muscles are innervated by the anterior rami of the **lower six intercostal nerves** (T7–12) and the **iliohypogastric** and **ilio-inguinal nerves** (L1).

XIII. The internal and external oblique muscles have a variety of functions which include:
- maintaining the tone of the abdominal wall;
- increasing abdominal pressure, e.g. during voiding;
- supporting the viscera;
- maintaining posture;
- lateral rotation of the trunk.

XIV. The conjoint tendon is the fused aponeuroses of the lower fibres of the **internal oblique** and **transversus abdominis muscles**. It passes medially to attach to the pubic crest and pectineal line, behind the superficial inguinal ring.

XV. The rectus sheath is a fibrous sheath enclosing the rectus abdominis muscles. The anterior layer of the sheath runs the length of the muscle, which extends from the fifth to seventh costal cartilages to the symphysis pubis and pubic crest. The posterior layer of the sheath is absent below a line approximately midway between the umbilicus and the pubis – the **arcuate line**. The anterior and posterior layers of the rectus sheath are structurally different above and below the arcuate line.

a. Above the line:
- **anterior layer** – consists of the aponeurosis of the external oblique and the anterior lamina on the internal oblique aponeurosis;
- **posterior layer** – consists of the posterior lamina of the internal oblique and the transversus abdominis aponeurosis.

b. Below the arcuate line:
- **anteriorly** – the aponeuroses of all three abdominal muscles pass anterior to the rectus abdominis;
- **posteriorly** – only the transversalis fascia separates the rectus abdominis from the parietal peritoneum.

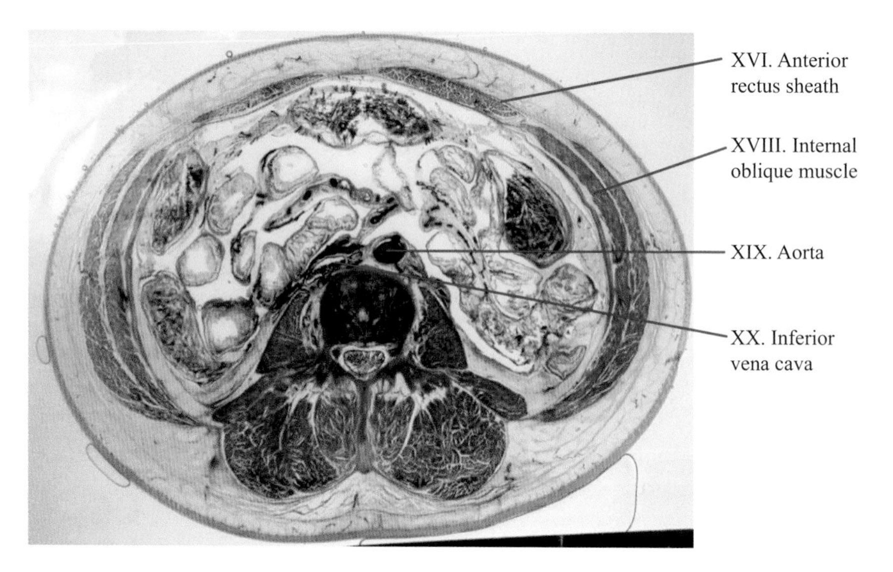

Image 6.2

XVI. The anterior rectus sheath lies anterior to the rectus abdominis muscle.

XVII. This slice is from **above** the arcuate line because the internal oblique aponeurosis splits to pass in front of and behind the rectus abdominis.

XVIII. The nerves and vessels run between the **transversus abdominis** and **internal oblique** muscles, much like the neurovascular plane in the thorax is between the inner two layers of muscles, i.e. the innermost intercostal and internal intercostal muscles.

XIX. The abdominal aorta lies just to the left of the midline, anterior to the lumbar vertebrae. It bifurcates at the level of L4.

XX. The IVC lies to the right of the lumbar vertebrae. It is formed at the level of L5.

XXI. The deep inguinal ring is most accurately described as lying just above the inguinal ligament within 1 cm either side of the **mid-inguinal point**, which is midway between the anterior superior iliac spine and the pubic symphysis. Note that multiple studies have now shown that this is a more accurate landmark than previous descriptions which sited it at the mid-point of the inguinal ligament (midway between the anterior superior iliac spine and the pubic tubercle).[3] Note also that the surface marking of the deep inguinal ring is the same as that for the femoral artery except that the deep ring is just above the inguinal ligament, whereas the femoral artery is just below. The deep ring is a 'defect' in the transversalis fascia, surrounded by the arching fibres of the transversus abdominis; it is larger in males.

XXII. The inguinal canal is an oblique intermuscular, slit-like passage above the inguinal ligament, transmitting the spermatic cord / round ligament and the ilio-inguinal nerve. It has the following boundaries:
- **anterior wall** – external oblique aponeurosis, reinforced laterally by the internal oblique muscle;
- **roof** – arching fibres of the internal oblique and transversus abdominis muscles;
- **posterior wall** – transversalis fascia, reinforced medially by the conjoint tendon;
- **floor** – the gutter-like inguinal ligament.

XXIII. Hesselbach's triangle,[4] or the inguinal triangle, has the following boundaries:
- **inferior** – medial half of the inguinal ligament
- **medial** – lower lateral border of the rectus abdominis
- **lateral** – (deep) inferior epigastric vessels.

XXIV. The clinical significance of the inguinal triangle is that direct inguinal hernias protrude directly through the abdominal wall within the triangle. This is readily apparent at laparoscopy. The position of an inguinal hernia in relation to the (deep) inferior epigastric vessels defines the nature of the hernia. Direct inguinal hernias emerge medial to the inferior epigastric vessels, whereas indirect inguinal hernias emerge lateral to the (deep) inferior epigastric vessels.

Question 2

I. The most likely diagnosis is a small bowel obstruction, possibly due to adhesions.

II. The small bowel consists of the duodenum, jejunum and ileum. The large bowel consists of the caecum, colon (ascending, transverse, descending and sigmoid), rectum and anal canal. They differ is several ways, as follows:

a. The large intestine has a larger calibre.

b. The large intestine is more fixed in position in comparison to the small intestine (the ascending and descending colon and rectum are retroperitoneal).

c. The large intestine has **taenia coli** – these are three longitudinal muscle bands running the length of the colon but not including the appendix. The small bowel does not have taenia coli but, instead, a complete circumferential outer layer of longitudinal muscle. The taenia coli broaden out to become a complete circumferential outer layer of longitudinal muscle at the rectum. Taenia are responsible for shortening the large bowel and contribute to the formation of haustra (sacculations).

d. The large bowel has **haustra** (sacculations) in part due to the presence of the taenia coli. They are not therefore visible in the small intestine. Their appearance on abdominal radiographs can be helpful in differentiating small and large bowel.

e. The small bowel contains **circular folds** (also known as plicae circulares or valvulae conniventes). These are found in the small intestine and are crescentic folds of mucosa projecting into the lumen, beginning a few centimetres beyond the pylorus and gradually disappearing in the terminal ileum. They act to slow the passage of intestinal contents and increase the absorptive capacity of the small bowel.

f. **Appendices epiploicae** are small adipose projections scattered over the free surface of the colon, becoming progressively more numerous towards the sigmoid colon. They are not found in the small intestine.

III. The average length of the small intestine at post-mortem is 6 m, but it is shorter *in vivo* because of muscle tone. There is no sharp distinction between the jejunum and the ileum, and arbitrarily the jejunum is stated to comprise the proximal two-fifths of the jejunoileal segment. Some general differences between the jejunum and ileum are as follows:

- The jejunum is located in the left upper infracolic compartment and centrally in the supine position; whereas the ileum tends to lie in the lower abdomen and pelvis.
- The jejunum is a slightly deeper red than the ileum on account of its greater vascularity.
- The jejunum has a slightly greater calibre than the ileum.
- The circular folds are more prominent and numerous in the jejunum. Their presence gives the jejunum a thicker appearance and feel, particularly more proximally.
- The small bowel mesentery becomes thicker and more 'fat laden' distally.
- The jejunum has fewer arterial arcades and longer vasa recta than the ileum. The mesenteric arcades in the ileal mesentery are more numerous, despite the ileum being less vascular than the jejunum.

IV. The duodenojejunal flexure is the junction between the fourth part of the duodenum and the beginning of the jejunum. The duodenum ends by ascending from the left side of the abdominal aorta to reach the inferior border of the pancreas at the level of the upper border of the L2 vertebra, where it turns abruptly anteriorly to join the jejunum. The duodenojejunal flexure is supported by a small suspensory muscle of the duodenum, also known as the ligament of Treitz.[5] The duodenojejunal flexure is an important landmark in the diagnosis of intestinal malrotation.

V. The duodenum is the shortest and most predictably positioned part of the small intestine. It has **four parts** and measures about 20–25 cm in length (the word duodenum is derived from the Latin for 12 because it is 12 fingerbreadths long).
   - First part (D1, superior) – this extends horizontally and to the right from the pylorus, lying anterior and lateral to the body of the L1 vertebra. It passes anterior to the common bile duct and portal vein and is approximately 5 cm long.
   - Second part (D2, descending) – this descends along the right side of the L2 and L3 vertebrae, forming a gentle curve embracing the head of the pancreas medially. It lies anterior to the hilum of the right kidney and its vasculature. The hepatic flexure is above and lateral. It receives bile and pancreatic juice via the major duodenal papilla on its medial wall. D2 is approximately 8 cm long.
   - Third part (D3, horizontal) – this passes medially from the right inferior border of L3 and crosses the inferior vena cava and aorta. The superior mesenteric vessels, transverse colon and the root of the small bowel mesentery all lie anterior. D3 is approximately 10 cm long.
   - Fourth part (D4, ascending) – see question IV above. The fourth part of the duodenum is approximately 2 cm long.

VI. **Yes**. The **first 2 cm of D1** has a mesentery. This dilated section of the duodenum is called the duodenal cap and is intraperitoneal. The rest of the duodenum is retroperitoneal.

VII. Chronic peptic ulcers are commonly found on the posterior aspect of the first part of the duodenum (in the duodenal cap). The gastroduodenal artery runs on the posterior surface of D1 and may be eroded by a penetrating ulcer, causing life-threatening gastrointestinal bleeding.

VIII. A represents the **cardia.** The cardia is the part of the stomach immediately adjacent to the gastro-oesophageal junction. It is histologically distinguishable by the presence of cardiac glands.

IX. B represents the **pylorus**, which consists of the wide pyloric antrum and narrower pyloric canal. A sphincter guards the distal pyloric canal and controls food discharging into the duodenum. The pyloric portion of the stomach can be histologically identified by the presence of pyloric glands.

X. C represents the **fundus** of the stomach, which is the superior part which is related to the left kidney and the left dome of the diaphragm. It readily distends with food, fluid and gas.

XI. The stomach is a foregut structure and is therefore supplied with arterial blood via the coeliac trunk. The lesser curvature is supplied by the **left** and **right gastric arteries**. The left gastric artery is usually a direct branch off the coeliac trunk; it initially ascends retroperitoneally before running forward in the upper part of the lesser omentum to reach the upper part of the lesser curvature. The right gastric artery is a branch of the hepatic artery; it runs forward from the posterior wall of the lesser sac into the lesser omentum near the lower part of the lesser curvature of the stomach.

XII. The blood supply to the pancreas is from both the coeliac trunk and the superior mesenteric artery, via the following branches:
- The **superior pancreaticoduodenal artery** is a branch of the gastroduodenal artery, which in turn is a branch of the common hepatic artery, which arises from the coeliac trunk. The superior pancreaticoduodenal artery supplies the head of the pancreas.
- The **inferior pancreaticoduodenal artery** is a branch of the superior mesenteric artery, or its first jejunal branch. It anastomoses with the superior pancreaticoduodenal artery to supply the head of the pancreas and the unicate process.
- There are also multiple pancreatic branches supplying the neck, body and tail of the pancreas, mostly arising from the **splenic artery**.

XIII. The pancreas is a retroperitoneal structure. The root of the transverse mesocolon crosses its anterior surface.

XIV. The pancreas has both endocrine and exocrine functions.
- **Endocrine** – less than 5% of the mass of the pancreas is responsible for its endocrine functions, mediated by the islets of Langerhans.[6] These cells are scattered through the substance of the pancreas and produce hormones such as insulin, glucagon, somatostatin, gastrin etc. which are involved in various metabolic cascades, including glucose metabolism.
- **Exocrine** – the remainder of the pancreas is involved in exocrine functions related to digestion. Exocrine cells are arranged in acini, which drain into intralobular ducts and then to the main pancreatic duct and ultimately the second part of the duodenum.

Question 3

I. Traditionally, the liver has been described as having **four anatomical lobes** – the left, right, caudate and quadrate lobes. They are separated by peritoneal attachments and ligaments. The falciform ligament and ligamentum venosum separate the left and right lobes. On the inferior surface of the liver, to the right of the ligamentum venosum, the porta hepatis separates the quadrate (anterior) and caudate (posterior) lobes.

II. Functionally the liver is split into left and right halves by an imaginary plane passing backwards from a line between the fundus of the gallbladder and the IVC (the principal plane). The quadrate lobe lies in the left functional half of the liver. The caudate lobe, which is developmentally distinct, is excluded from this division. Each 'hemiliver' has its own branch of the portal vein, bile duct and hepatic artery. The hepatic veins are distributed differently (see below).

III. The left and right functional halves of the liver are each further divided into **functional liver segments**. There are eight segments in total. Each segment has an independent blood supply from the portal vein and hepatic arteries, and independent biliary drainage. The left hemiliver comprises segments II–IV (segment IV being the equivalent of the quadrate lobe), and the right hemiliver segments V to VIII. Segment I is separate and corresponds to the anatomical caudate lobe.

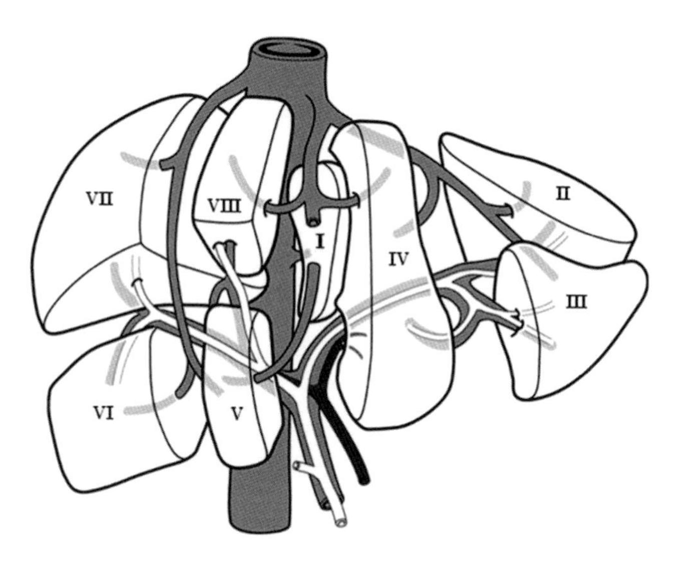

Image 6.3 **Liver segments**

IV. Knowledge of the segmental structure of the liver helps the hepatobiliary surgeon minimise blood loss during liver resection. It has also contributed dramatically to liver transplantation, facilitating split-liver transplantation and living donor liver transplantation. The liver is capable of regeneration (although regenerated liver does not form functional segments), and up to 80% of the liver can be removed safely provided the remnant is healthy; the remnant regenerates the liver to almost its original size within three months.

V. The liver is supplied by two principal routes:
   a. The **portal vein** brings deoxygenated blood from the abdominal part of the digestive system and contributes to approximately 70% of the hepatic blood supply.

b. The **hepatic artery**, a branch of the coeliac trunk, provides the liver with oxygenated blood and constitutes approximately 30% of the hepatic blood supply.

VI. The hepatic artery and portal vein, along with the bile duct, are collectively known as the *portal triad*. The portal triad runs within the free edge of the lesser omentum (also known as the **hepatoduodenal ligament**), which also forms the anterior boundary of the epiploic foramen (the entrance to the lesser sac). The portal vein lies posterior, the hepatic artery anterior and to the left, and the bile duct anterior to the right. Lymphatic vessels and autonomic nerves also run with the portal triad.

VII. The **Pringle manoeuvre**[7] involves compressing the portal triad in the free edge of the lesser omentum to temporarily control the inflow of blood to the liver. This assists the surgeon with identification and repair of the cause of the bleeding from branches of the hepatic artery or portal vein.

VIII. There are **three main hepatic veins**: right, left and middle. Importantly, they have no extrahepatic course, passing directly from the liver parenchyma into the IVC just below the diaphragm. The middle hepatic vein travels in the principal plane of the liver, and the right and left hepatic veins drain the right and left functional halves of the liver. The hepatic veins do not respect the boundaries of the functional segments. The caudate lobe drains independently into the IVC via several small short veins.

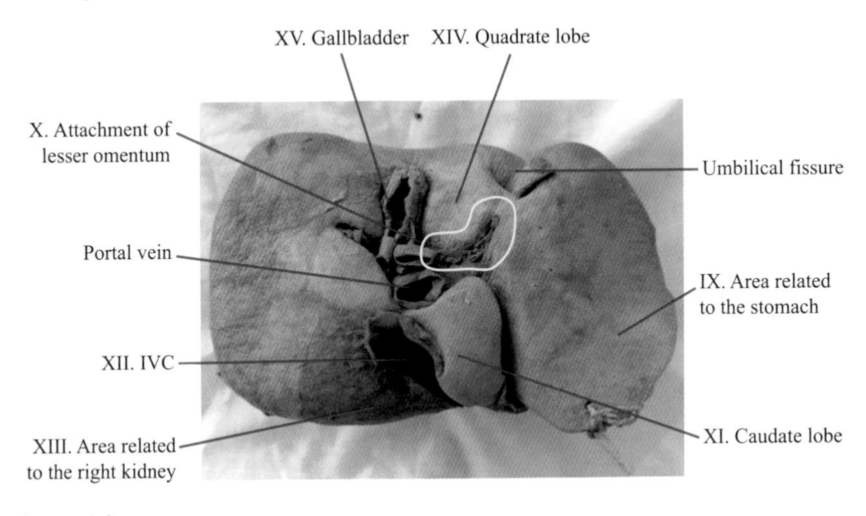

Image 6.4

IX. The undersurface of the left lobe of the liver is related to the anterior aspect of the fundus and body of the stomach.

X. The lesser omentum is a double peritoneal fold which runs from the lesser curve of the stomach and proximal duodenum (D1) to the undersurface of the liver. It attaches to the liver in an L-shape, along the line of the ligamentum venosum and across to encircle the porta hepatis.

XI. The caudate lobe is located adjacent to the IVC. It is the only part of the liver lying within the lesser sac. The caudate process, which runs between the IVC and porta hepatis on the undersurface of the liver, forms the roof of the epiploic foramen.

XII. The retrohepatic IVC is half embedded within the liver substance, partially overlapped by the caudate lobe. It receives the three major hepatic veins just below the diaphragm as it exits the liver superiorly.

XIII. The **right** kidney and right suprarenal gland are related to the postero-inferior surface of the right lobe of the liver in the region of the bare area, which has no peritoneal covering.

XIV. The quadrate lobe of the liver lies between the gallbladder fossa and the ligamentum teres running in the free lower margin of the falciform ligament and the umbilical fissure in the liver.

XV. The gallbladder is a pear-shaped organ that lies in the gallbladder fossa. The gallbladder fundus is completely surrounded by peritoneum which binds the body and neck of the gallbladder to the undersurface of the right lobe of the liver.

XVI. The **cystic artery** supplies the gallbladder and cystic duct. It normally arises from the right hepatic artery which typically passes *behind* the common hepatic duct. Both the origin and course of the cystic artery may vary.

Question 4

I. The **abdominal aorta** in this CT scan is aneurysmal and has a thin rim of calcification. The lumen of the aorta is patent, with vascular contrast within it. There does not appear to be extravasation of contrast from the aorta.

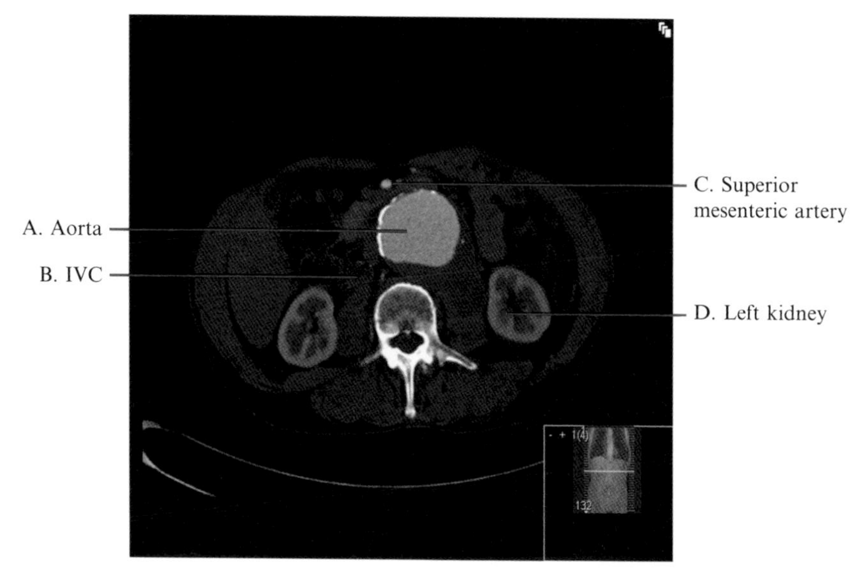

Image 6.5

II. The **inferior vena cava** lies in close proximity to the right side of the aorta. A potential complication of a ruptured abdominal aortic aneurysm (AAA) (or after its repair) is the formation of an aorto-caval fistula.
III. This is the **superior mesenteric artery.**
IV. This is the **left kidney.**

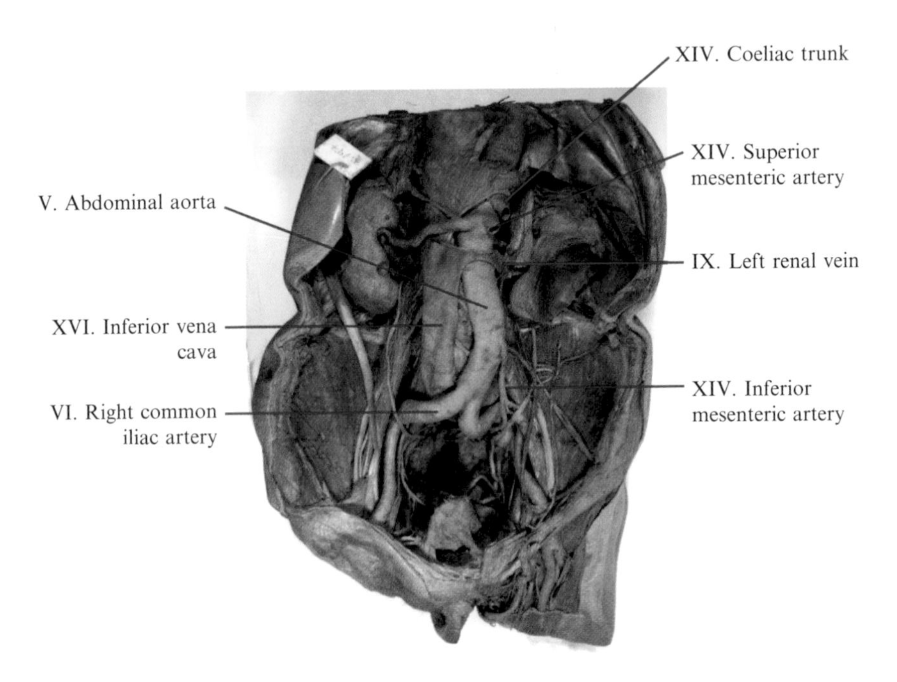

Image 6.6

V. See Image 6.6.
VI. See Image 6.6.
VII. The abdominal aorta bifurcates into the two common iliac arteries at the level of the **L4 vertebra.** It enters the abdomen by passing through the aortic hiatus at the level of T12. It descends anterior to the lumbar spine, slightly to the left of the midline.
VIII. The tips of the iliac crests lie in the **supracristal plane** at the level of the L4 vertebra, which corresponds to the level of the bifurcation of the abdominal aorta. This is just below and to the left of the umbilicus in a non-obese individual.
IX. The renal veins lie anterior to the renal arteries.
X. The renal arteries normally arise from the abdominal aorta at the **L2** vertebral level, the right often slightly higher than the left, at the level of L1.

XI. The **right renal artery** is longer than the left and normally passes behind the following structures:
- IVC;
- right renal vein;
- head of the pancreas;
- second part of the duodenum.

The left renal artery passes behind the following structures:
- left renal vein;
- splenic vein;
- body of the pancreas.

XII. The abdominal aorta is crossed anteriorly by the **body of the pancreas**; the renal arteries also arise at this level. Other anterior relations of the abdominal aorta, from superior to inferior, include:
- the coeliac plexus and lesser sac, which lie between the aorta and the left lobe of the liver;
- the body of the pancreas, with the splenic vein on its posterior surface;
- the left renal vein, which itself is crossed by the superior mesenteric artery;
- the third part of the duodenum and uncinate process of the pancreas;
- the oblique origin of the small intestinal mesentery.

XIII. The aorta has three unpaired anterior branches. These are the following:

a. The **coeliac trunk**. This arises at the level of T12, just below the level of the aortic hiatus. It usually has three branches: the left gastric, common hepatic and splenic arteries. The coeliac trunk supplies foregut structures.

b. The **superior mesenteric artery**. This originates approximately 1 cm distal to the coeliac trunk, at the level of L1. It supplies the midgut (distal second part of duodenum to distal transverse colon).

c. The **inferior mesenteric artery**. This is the lowest and smallest of the three anterior branches, arising at the level of the L3 vertebra. It supplies the hindgut.

The aorta has one unpaired posterior branch, the median sacral artery, which arises a little above the bifurcation of the aorta, at the level of L4.

XIV. The coeliac trunk is visible just below the aortic hiatus and just above the superior mesenteric artery.

XV. The marginal artery, or artery of Drummond,[8] runs in the mesentery of the large bowel parallel to the colon. It is fed by branches from both the superior and inferior mesenteric arteries. When the IMA is occluded following an EVAR, the SMA can usually perfuse the hindgut adequately via the marginal artery.

XVI. See Image 6.6.

XVII. The IVC is formed by the union of the common iliac veins, at the level of **L5**, just to the right of the midline. It ascends through the abdomen to the right of the aorta, on the psoas major muscle. It is stated to pass through the central tendon of the diaphragm at the level of T8, after which it enters the right atrium.

XVIII. The major tributaries of the IVC are the:
- common iliac veins;
- third and fourth lumbar veins;
- right gonadal vein – the left gonadal vein drains to the left renal vein;
- renal veins;
- right suprarenal vein – the left suprarenal vein usually drains to the left renal vein;
- inferior phrenic veins;
- hepatic veins.

Question 5

I. Scenarios of patients who are shocked, whether after trauma or following postoperative complications, are common in the MRCS examinations. You should be familiar with a structured answer based on algorithms learnt on ATLS® (Advanced Trauma Life Support) and CCrISP® courses. For example:

This patient should be managed as per ATLS guidelines. His airway should be cleared and his C-spine controlled. His breathing should be assessed and the patient started on high-flow oxygen. He is hypotensive and tachycardic and therefore shocked. Given he has sustained abdominal trauma, this is likely to be grade III hypovolaemic shock. I would begin aggressive fluid resuscitation with intravenous crystalloids and blood through two wide-bore cannulas.

II. Left-sided shoulder tip pain after splenic rupture is caused by irritation of the undersurface of the diaphragm from blood in the peritoneal cavity. The pain is referred to the C3–5 dermatomes in the shoulder region via the phrenic nerve, which is sensory to the central region of the diaphragm. This is known as **Kehr's sign.**[9]

III. The spleen is supplied exclusively by the **splenic artery**, a branch of the coeliac trunk. The splenic artery has a tortuous course, running behind the upper border of the pancreas, anterior to the left kidney and suprarenal gland, before entering the splenorenal ligament to reach the hilum of the spleen. It also supplies parts of the pancreas and stomach. It divides into two or three main branches before entering the hilum of the spleen, where the branches further divide into four or five segmental arteries.

IV. The spleen has fairly mobile peritoneal attachments and is therefore at risk of rotational and deceleration injuries which may rupture the parenchyma or tear the splenic vessels. In addition, the splenic capsule is thin and may rupture following trauma, which includes traction on peritoneal ligaments or adhesions at surgery. Splenic injury causes haemorrhage into the abdominal cavity.

V. The spleen is located on the left side of the abdomen, beneath the 9–11th ribs, with its long axis in the line of the 10th rib. It extends from a point about 5 cm to the left of the midline at the level of the 10th thoracic vertebra as far as the midaxillary line. In healthy adults, the spleen is not normally palpable below the costal margin.

VI. The inferomedial 'visceral' surface of the spleen has several important relations:
- **Stomach** – the anteromedial aspect of the spleen lies adjacent to the posterior part of the fundus, body and greater curvature of the stomach.
- **Left kidney** – the inferomedial aspect of the spleen is related to the left kidney.
- **Splenic flexure** – the inferior pole of the spleen is related to the splenic flexure and phrenicocolic ligament.
- **Pancreas** – the tail of the pancreas may extend into the splenorenal ligament and come into contact with the spleen at its hilum. The tail of the pancreas is at risk of injury when ligating the splenic vessels during a splenectomy.

Question 6

I. The most likely diagnosis is **ureteric colic**. Note that the commonly used term 'renal colic' is wrongly applied to a calculus within a ureter. An important diagnosis to rule out, is a leaking AAA, which may present with similar symptoms.

II. The ureter is approximately 3 mm in diameter but narrower at several sites including:
- at its origin, the junction between the renal pelvis and the ureter;
- at the pelvic brim;
- at its termination, the ureteric orifice (the narrowest segment).

A calculus is most likely to become impacted at any of these sites.

III. To be able to make sense of the landmarks it is important to know the normal anatomy of the ureter. Each ureter leaves the kidney and descends through the abdomen on the medial edge of the psoas major muscle, which therefore separates the ureter from the tips of the transverse processes of the lumbar vertebrae. The right ureter is crossed by the second part of the duodenum, and the right gonadal, right colic and ileocolic vessels. The left ureter is crossed by the left colic and left gonadal vessels. The ureter passes anterior to the bifurcation of the common iliac artery and enters the pelvic brim anterior to the sacroiliac joint. The pelvic ureters then descend anterior to the internal iliac arteries, towards the ischial spine, where they turn medially to enter the base of the bladder. Landmarks on an abdominal radiograph include:
- just medial to the tips of the transverse processes of the lumbar vertebrae;

- sacroiliac joints, at the pelvic brim;
- ischial spines;
- pubic tubercle (a rough projection of the ureterovesical junction).

A radio-opaque calculus may be seen along this course.

IV. Ureters have a rich blood supply from several arteries which anastomose along its length. When the ureter is severed, it usually heals well after repair. The arterial sources of supply include:
- renal arteries
- gonadal arteries
- common and internal iliac arteries
- vesical arteries
- uterine arteries
- abdominal aorta.

V. Both ureters enter the base of the bladder posteriorly. They pass obliquely through the wall of the bladder for 1–2 cm before terminating at the slit-like ureteric orifices, which are at the upper lateral corners of the **trigone.** Their oblique passage through the wall of the bladder helps to prevent vesicoureteric reflux during bladder emptying. When the bladder is empty the orifices are approximately 2.5 cm apart, and when full they are approximately 5 cm apart.

VI. The bladder wall has three layers, as follows:

a. **Mucosa** – lined by urothelium which is a transitional epithelium. The latter lines most of the urinary tract, from the renal pelvis to the proximal urethra and also the prostatic ducts and ductus deferens. Malignant change results in transitional cell carcinoma.

b. **Smooth muscle**, or the 'detrusor coat'.

c. **Adventitia** containing connective tissue. Superiorly this also includes the peritoneum, which is reflected onto the dome of the bladder from the anterior abdominal wall.

VII. In men, the posterior relations of the bladder are the:
- rectovesical pouch
- seminal vesicles and ductus deferens
- rectum.

NB: the ductus deferens crosses from lateral to medial above the ureter in the male pelvis.

VIII. In women the bladder is posteriorly related to the anterior wall of the vagina and the vesicouterine pouch.

IX. The male urethra is around 20 cm long and has several parts:
- **Preprostatic urethra**, about 1 cm long between the base of the bladder and the prostate. This section of the male urethra is surrounded by circular smooth muscle continuous with the neck of the bladder, forming a preprostatic sphincter, which prevents retrograde ejaculation (and provides some degree of continence when the external urethral sphincter is damaged). It is commonly damaged during transurethral resection of the prostate.

- **Prostatic urethra**, 3–4 cm long. The ejaculatory and prostatic ducts discharge into this section which has a midline ridge posteriorly, the urethral crest. An elevation on this crest, the verumontanum, is an important surgical landmark during transurethral resection of the prostate. The distal segment of the prostatic urethra is immobile due to the attachment of the puboprostatic ligament.
- **Membranous urethra**, 2 cm. The membranous urethra is narrow (the narrowest segment after the external urethral orifice) and is surrounded by the voluntary external urethral sphincter (striated muscle).
- **Spongy urethra**, about 15 cm long. This can be subdivided into the bulbar urethra, the widest part of the urethra surrounded by the bulbospongiosus muscle, and the penile component which is contained within the corpus spongiosum of the penis and opens at the external urethral meatus.

X. The preprostatic and prostatic parts of the urethra are lined with the same urothelium as the bladder. **Distal to the ejaculatory ducts**, the urethral epithelium becomes stratified columnar in type (containing mucus-secreting cells), and the very terminal urethra is lined by stratified squamous epithelium.

ENDNOTES

1 Charles McBurney (1845–1913), American surgeon.
2 Terence Jenkins (1913–2007), British surgeon.
3 If you want to read more, consult Hale SJ, Mirjalili SA, Stringer MD. Inconsistencies in surface anatomy: the need for an evidence-based reappraisal. *Clin Anat* 2010;23(8):922–30.
4 Franz Hesselbach (1759–1816), German surgeon and anatomist.
5 Václav Treitz (1819–1872), Czech pathologist.
6 Paul Langerhans (1847–1888), German pathologist.
7 James Pringle (1863–1941), Australian-born British surgeon.
8 Sir David Drummond (1852–1932), English physician.
9 Johannes Otto Kehr (1862–1916), German surgeon (attribution controversial).

7

Head and neck questions

Question 1

Scenario:
A patient presents with a lump in the posterior triangle of her neck. You are asked to examine the patient.

I. What are the boundaries of the posterior triangle of the neck?
II. What are the boundaries of the anterior triangle of the neck?
III. What are the attachments of the sternocleidomastoid muscle?
IV. What is the function of the sternocleidomastoid muscle?
V. What vein crosses the sternocleidomastoid muscle superficially?
VI. What are the surface markings of this vein?
VII. What does the spinal accessory nerve innervate?
VIII. What are the approximate surface markings of the spinal accessory nerve?
IX. List some causes of a lump within the posterior triangle of the neck.
X. Why is the sixth cervical vertebra (C6) an important vertebral level in the neck?
XI. At what vertebral level is the hyoid bone?
XII. What muscles attach to the hyoid bone?

With regards to Image 7.1:

XIII. Identify the sternocleidomastoid muscle.
XIV. What is its innervation?
XV. Identify the sternohyoid muscle.
XVI. Identify the omohyoid muscle.
XVII. What other two muscles belong to the infrahyoid (strap) group of muscles?
XVIII. What is the innervation of these four muscles, and what are their functions?

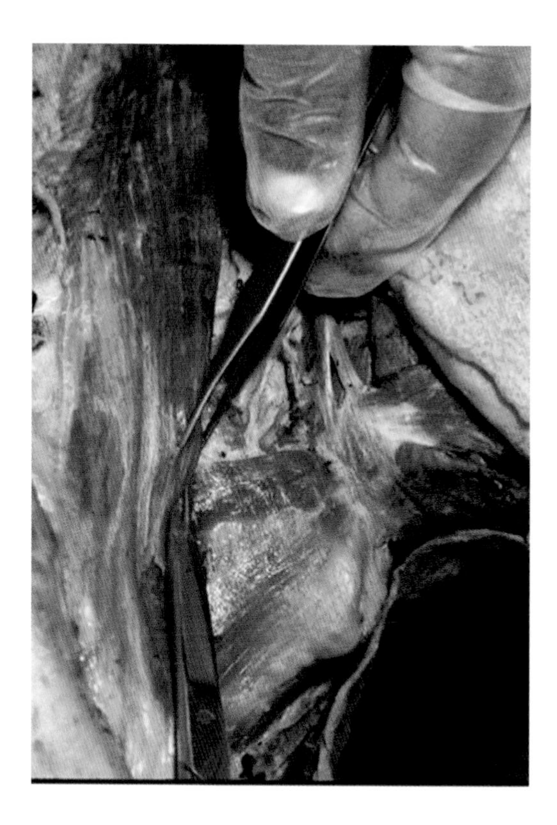

Image 7.1

Whilst examining this patient, you are urgently called away to assist the anaesthetist with another patient with acute airway obstruction – the anaesthetist is unable to intubate and ventilate a patient with a severe anaphylactic reaction. You elect to perform a cricothyroidotomy.

XIX. What are the anatomical landmarks for this procedure?

You achieve a secure airway in the patient and you would like to gain central venous access.

XX. What are the surface landmarks of the internal jugular vein?
XXI. What are the surface landmarks for subclavian vein cannulation?

Question 2

Scenario:

A patient with thyroid cancer is due to have a total thyroidectomy. Your consultant asks you to read up on the anatomy of the thyroid gland and pay particular attention to the nerves and vessels supplying the gland.

I. How many lobes does the thyroid have and what joins the lobes?
II. Where is the thyroid gland positioned in relation to the cervical vertebrae?
III. What fascial layer encloses the gland?

IV. What are the posterior relations of the thyroid gland?
V. What arteries, encountered during the thyroidectomy, will need to be ligated?
VI. What veins would need to be ligated?
VII. Which nerve(s) lying in close proximity to the gland are at risk of injury during a thyroidectomy?
VIII. What steps can be taken intraoperatively to minimise the risk of injuring nerves?
IX. What would be the effects of injury to the nerve(s) supplying the thyroid gland?
X. What types of cells make up the thyroid gland?
XI. What types of cancers may arise from these cells, and what is their likely mode of metastatic spread?
XII. What other endocrine organ(s) closely related to the thyroid gland could potentially be injured by thyroidectomy?

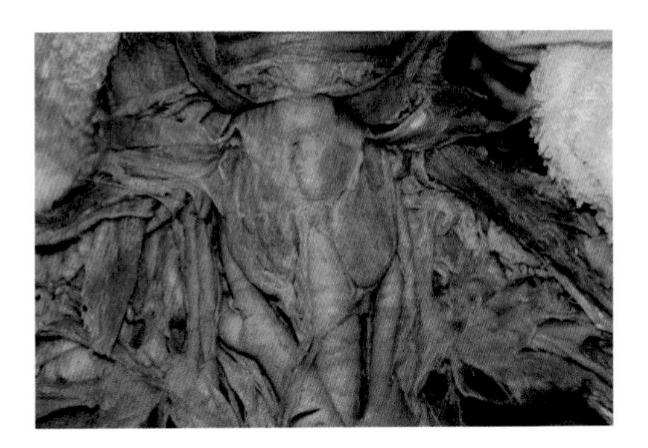

Image 7.2

With regards to Image 7.2:
XIII. Identify the:
- lobes of the thyroid
- trachea
- inferior thyroid veins.

Question 3

Scenario:

A patient presents with a lump over his jaw.

I. What are the surface markings of the parotid gland?
II. What are the surface markings of the parotid duct?
III. What structures pass through the gland?

With regards to Image 7.3:
IV. Identify structure A.
V. Identify the structure labelled B. What is its function?

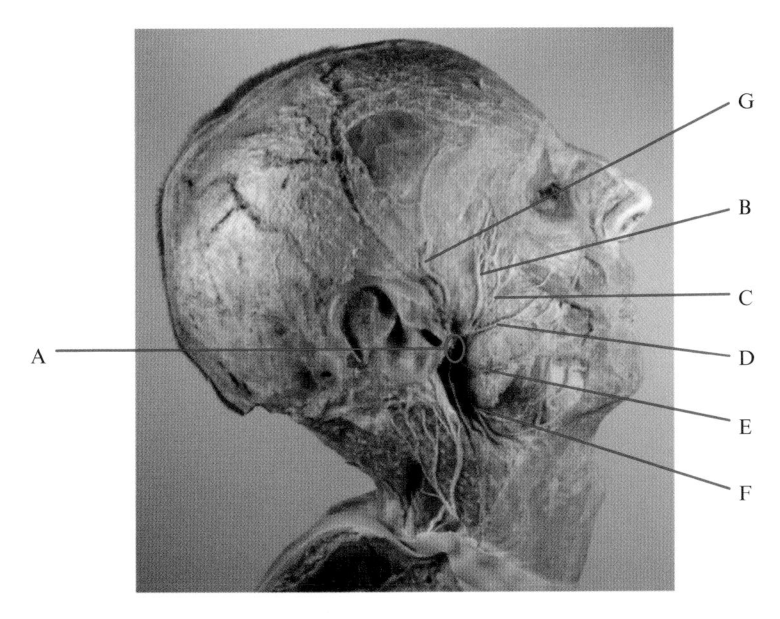

Image 7.3

VI. Identify the structure labelled C. What is its function?
VII. Identify the structure labelled D. What is its function?
VIII. Identify the structure labelled E. What is its function?
IX. Identify the structure labelled F. What is its function?
X. Identify structure G. When might this structure be biopsied?
XI. What is the differential diagnosis of a lump or swelling in the parotid gland?
XII. How many lobes does the submandibular salivary gland have, and what structure distinguishes them?
XIII. Where is the orifice of the submandibular duct?
XIV. What nerve is most at risk during a surgical approach to the submandibular gland?
XV. What would be the effect of an injury to this nerve?

Question 4

Scenario:
A patient is referred to the surgical team for a vascular opinion following a transient ischaemic attack (TIA).
With regards to the CT angiogram in Image 7.4:

I. Identify A.
II. At what level does it bifurcate?
III. Identify B.
IV. What are its terminal branches?
V. Identify C; how many branches does structure C have in the neck?
VI. What is the first branch of C?

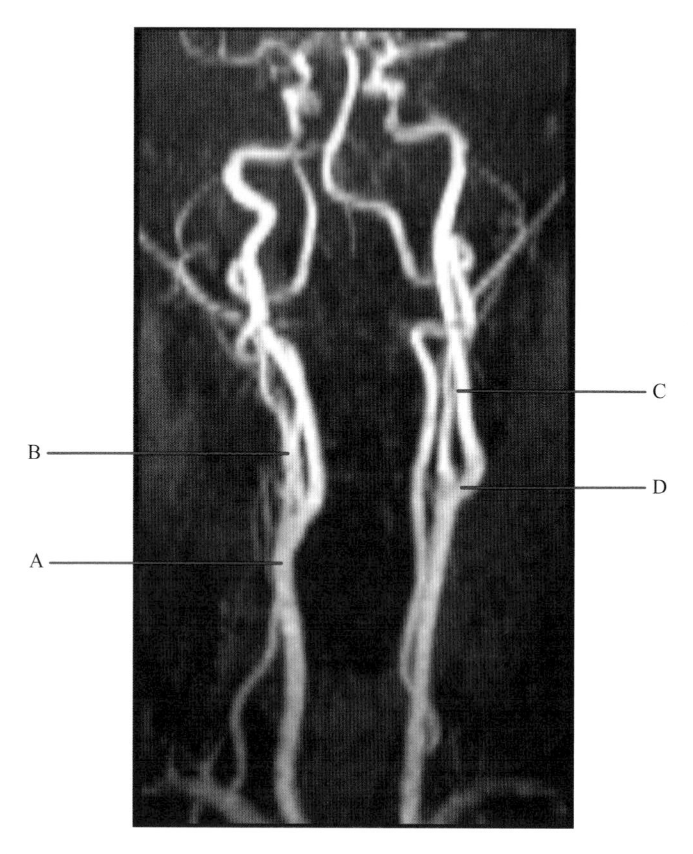

Image 7.4

VII. What is the localised dilation, labelled D?
VIII. What is its function?
IX. What fascia surrounds A?
X. What other structures are enclosed within this fascial layer?
XI. From which artery does A originate?
XII. If this patient underwent a carotid endarterectomy, what nerves would be at risk of injury?

A young man presents with pain, numbness and tingling in the upper limb and is suspected of having a 'thoracic outlet syndrome'.

With regards to Image 7.5:

XIII. Identify structure A.
XIV. Identify structure B.
XV. Identify structure C.
XVI. What nerve supplies this structure?
XVII. What part of the brachial plexus does D represent?
XVIII. Identify structure E.
XIX. What is the thoracic outlet?
XX. What is meant by thoracic outlet obstruction syndrome?

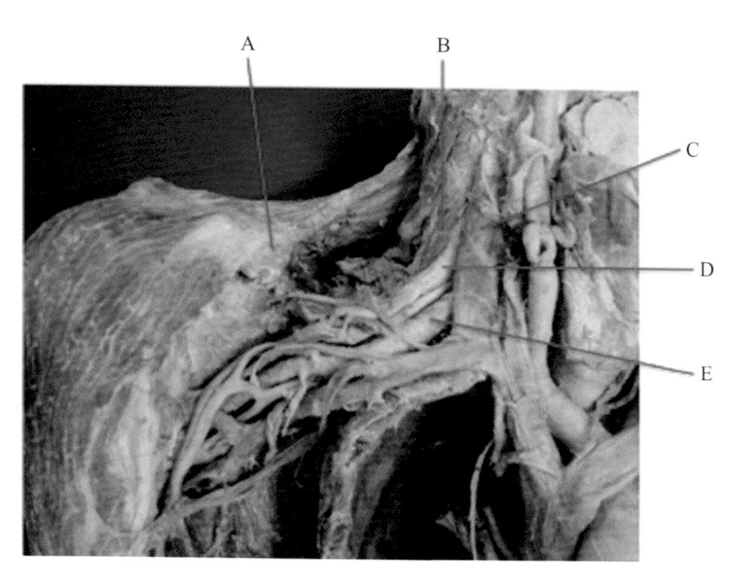

Image 7.5

Question 5

Scenario:
You are performing a diagnostic laryngoscopy on a patient.

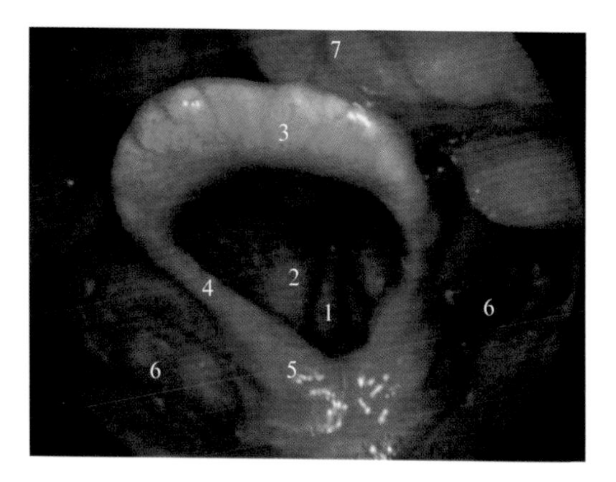

Image 7.6 http://commons.wikimedia.org/wiki/File%3aLarynx_normal.jpg

With regards to Image 7.6:

I. What is structure 1?
II. What muscle is responsible for abducting the vocal cord?
III. What nerve supplies this muscle?

IV. What is structure 2?
V. What is structure 3?
VI. What is the function of structure 3 during deglutition?
VII. What is structure 4?
VIII. What is structure 5?
IX. What are the structures labelled 6?
X. What nerve lies deep to the mucous membrane of 6?
XI. What is structure 7?

Question 6

Scenario:
You are teaching medical students the anatomy of the base of the skull.

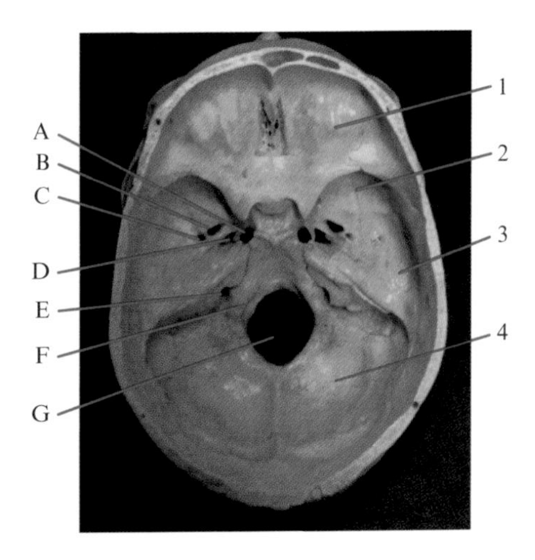

Image 7.7

With regards to Image 7.7, name the foramina labelled as structures A to G, and describe the items that pass through them:

I. Structure A.
II. Structure B.
III. Structure C.
IV. Structure D.
V. Structure E.
VI. Structure F.
VII. What is the function of the nerve that leaves the skull through foramen F?
VIII. Structure G.

Identify the bones labelled 1–4:

IX. Bone 1.
X. Bone 2.
XI. Bone 3.
XII. Bone 4.
XIII. How would you assess the sensory and motor function of the trigeminal nerve?

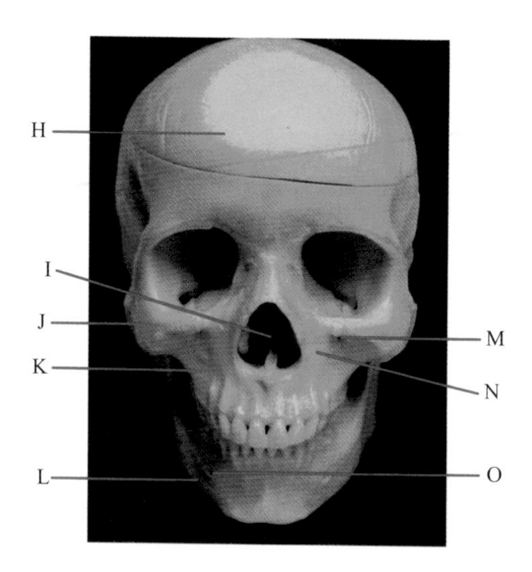

Image 7.8

With regards to Image 7.8, identify the following structures:

XIV. Structure H.
XV. Structure I.
XVI. Structure J.
XVII. Structure K.
XVIII. Structure L.
XIX. What foramen is indicated by M and what passes through it?
XX. Which artery ascends in the region of the nasolabial fold?
XXI. What foramen is indicated by O and what passes through it?

8

Head and neck answers

Question 1

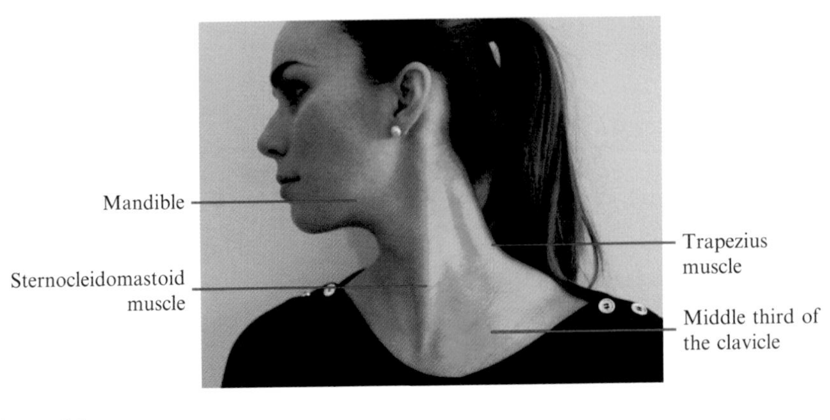

Image 8.1

I. Each side of the neck is divided into anterior and posterior triangles by the obliquely running sternocleidomastoid (SCM) muscle. The posterior triangle of the neck has the following borders:
   - **anterior border** – posterior border of SCM
   - **posterior border** – anterior border of trapezius
   - **inferior border** – middle third of the clavicle
   - **roof** – investing layer of deep cervical fascia
   - **floor** – prevertebral fascia with underlying musculature.

   The posterior triangle is spiralised so that its apex is at the superior nuchal line of the occipital bone, 4–5 cm medial to the mastoid process. The contents of the triangle include the accessory nerve, lymph nodes, the inferior belly of omohyoid, the transverse cervical and suprascapular arteries, and branches of the cervical plexus. The third part of the subclavian artery and the lower part of the external jugular vein just creep into the corner of the triangle anteriorly behind where the SCM inserts into the clavicle.

II. The anterior triangle of the neck is more complicated than the posterior. The borders of this inverted triangle are:
- **anterior border** – the midline of the neck
- **posterior border** – anterior border of the SCM
- **base** – inferior border of the mandible and angle of mandible to mastoid process
- **apex** – suprasternal notch
- **roof** – platysma and associated subcutaneous tissue.

The digastric and omohyoid muscles subdivide the anterior triangle into:
- an unpaired submental triangle bordered by the diverging anterior bellies of the digastric muscles;
- three paired triangles: the submandibular, carotid and muscular triangles.

The anterior triangle can also be divided by the hyoid bone into suprahyoid and infrahyoid regions.

III. The SCM has two heads:
- **sternal head** – arises from the anterior aspect of the manubrium
- **clavicular head** – arises from the medial third of the clavicle.

The muscle is inserted into the mastoid process and adjacent superior nuchal line of the occipital bone.

IV. The SCM is a powerful muscle with many functions. Acting alone it rotates or laterally flexes the neck (the ear approaches the ipsilateral shoulder and the chin rotates to the opposite side). Acting with its counterpart, it flexes the neck. It also acts as an accessory muscle of respiration by lifting the sternum.

V. The **external jugular vein** is formed by the union of the posterior branch of the retromandibular vein and the posterior auricular vein. The vein crosses the SCM muscle from medial to lateral as it descends through the superficial fascia of the neck. Approximately 2 cm above the clavicle it pierces the deep cervical fascia to empty into the subclavian vein. It is readily seen during a Valsalva manoeuvre.

VI. The surface marking of the external jugular vein can be represented by a line drawn from the angle of the mandible to the clavicle at the posterior border of the SCM.

VII. The spinal accessory nerve (CN XI) has only motor fibres. It innervates both the **sternocleidomastoid** and **trapezius** muscles.

VIII. The surface marking of the spinal accessory nerve within the posterior triangle is not really reliable because of variations in the course and branching pattern of the nerve. However, for exam purposes, it would be reasonable to state that it enters the posterior triangle of the neck approximately halfway down the posterior border of the SCM, and leaves the triangle by piercing the anterior border of the trapezius about 3–5 cm above the clavicle.

IX. The contents of the posterior triangle of the neck are numerous (see part I above), and therefore the differential diagnosis is lengthy. However, one way of answering this question is to base it on the anatomy, emphasising the commonest cause first:
- lymphadenopathy (benign or malignant)
- lymphangioma (cystic hygroma)
- superficial lesions – lipomas, sebaceous cysts etc.
- pharyngeal pouch
- cervical rib
- subclavian artery aneurysm.

X. The sixth cervical vertebra is an important anatomical level in the neck because it is an approximate guide to the following structures:
- The cricoid cartilage.
- Vessels:
  - the inferior thyroid artery and middle thyroid vein enter and exit the thyroid;
  - the vertebral artery enters the transverse foramen;
  - the level at which the common carotid artery can be compressed against the transverse process of C6.
- Viscera:
  - junction between the pharynx and oesophagus;
  - junction between the larynx and trachea.
- Nerves:
  - level of the middle cervical sympathetic ganglion.
- Muscles:
  - level at which the superior belly of omohyoid crosses the carotid sheath.

XI. The U-shaped hyoid bone lies at the level of the **C3** vertebra.

XII. The hyoid bone has a large number of muscles attaching to it, which contribute to the tongue, floor of the mouth, epiglottis, pharynx and larynx. These muscles include the following:
- **Suprahyoid muscles** – mylohyoid, geniohyoid, stylohyoid and digastric. The digastric actually inserts indirectly via an intermediate tendon which attaches to the body and greater horn of the hyoid bone.
- **Infrahyoid muscles** – sternohyoid and omohyoid are superficial with thyrohyoid deep to them. Note that the fourth infrahyoid muscle is the sternothyroid which is attached to the manubrium and thyroid cartilage.
- **Other muscles** – middle pharyngeal constrictor and the hyoglossus.

XIII. For more information on SCM, refer back to parts (III) and (IV) of this question.

XIV. The SCM muscle receives motor fibres from the spinal accessory nerve (CN XI). Proprioception is conveyed by branches from the cervical plexus (C2/3).

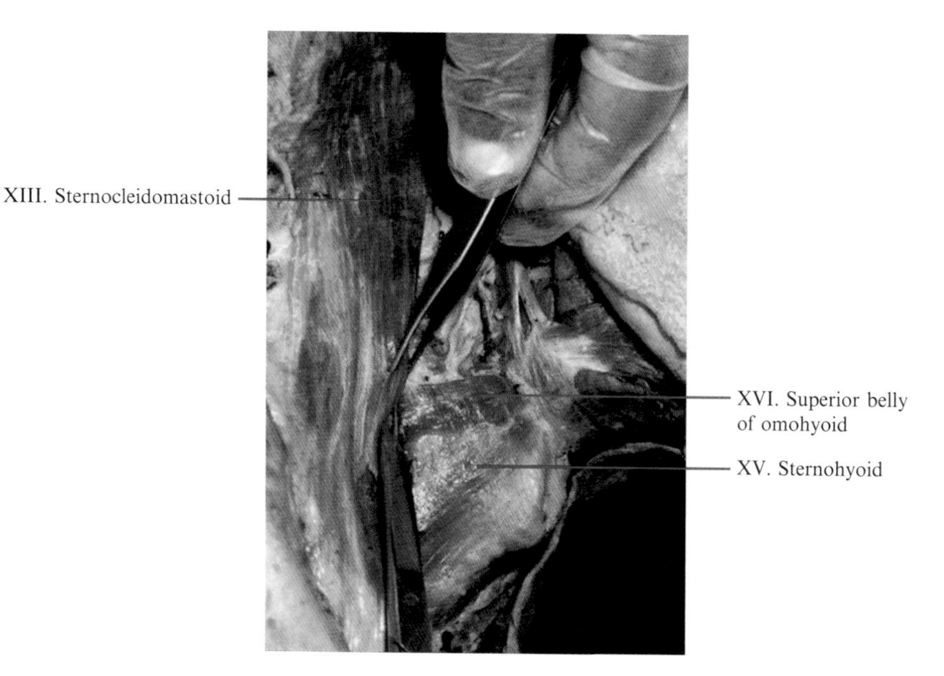

Image 8.2

XV. As its name suggests, the **sternohyoid** attaches to the sternum and hyoid.

XVI. **Omohyoid** has a superior and inferior belly, joined by a central tendon. The superior belly originates from the hyoid bone lateral to the origin of sternohyoid. The inferior belly originates from the upper scapula near the scapular notch. The central tendon varies in length and crosses the internal jugular vein; it is connected to the clavicle and first rib by a fascial sling.

XVII. The other two infrahyoid muscles are the **sternothyroid** and **thyrohyoid** muscles. Sternothyroid, deep to the sternohyoid muscle, extends between the manubrium and the oblique line on the thyroid cartilage. Thyrohyoid, also deep to sternohyoid, passes cranially from the oblique line on the lamina of the thyroid cartilage to the greater cornu of the hyoid bone.

XVIII. The innervation and actions of the four infrahyoid muscles, two superficial and two deep, are shown in Table 8.1.

XIX. A cricothyroidotomy is performed by inserting an airway through the **cricothyroid membrane** into the trachea (in the midline). The cricothyroid membrane lies between the thyroid cartilage (at the level of C4) and the cricoid cartilage (at the level of C6).

XX. The internal jugular vein is the most common site for placing a central venous catheter. The 'textbook' definition of the landmarks where a needle should be inserted during cannulation of the internal jugular vein is as follows:

- The apex of a triangle formed between the sternal and clavicular heads of the sternocleidomastoid and the clavicle.
- The needle should then be directed:
  - caudally
  - angled 30° posteriorly
  - aiming towards the ipsilateral nipple.

Anatomical considerations during this procedure include the relationship of nearby structures to the internal jugular vein: common carotid artery medially, vagus nerve and sympathetic trunk posteriorly, and the domes of the pleura and thoracic duct (left side only) inferiorly.

Table 8.1

Muscle	Innervation	Actions
Sternohyoid	Ansa cervicalis (C1–3)	Depress the larynx (sternothyroid) or hyoid bone (sternohyoid, omohyoid and thyrohyoid) after it has been elevated e.g. in swallowing. When the hyoid is stabilised, thyrohyoid can elevate the larynx (e.g. when singing high notes)
Omohyoid	Ansa cervicalis (C1–3)	
Sternothyroid	Ansa cervicalis (C2–3)	
Thyrohyoid	C1 fibres hitch-hiking on the hypoglossal nerve	

XXI. Subclavian central lines are now less commonly used in elective settings. This is in part due to their intimate relationship to the pleura, with the increased risk of causing an iatrogenic pneumothorax, and because of the inability to provide manual compression of the subclavian artery behind the clavicle if it is inadvertently punctured. When placing a subclavian line, the landmarks for needle insertion are as follows:

- The junction between the middle and medial thirds of the clavicle.
- The needle should then be directed:
  - posteriorly behind the clavicle
  - slightly cephalad
  - aiming towards the suprasternal notch.

Question 2

I. The thyroid gland is made up of **two lateral lobes** joined by an isthmus. Each lobe is conical in shape, with its apex pointing cephalad. Occasionally a **pyramidal lobe** projects up towards the hyoid bone, usually from the isthmus.

II. The normally placed thyroid gland lies between the level of the C5 and T1 vertebrae. The isthmus overlies the second and third tracheal rings, and each lobe extends from below the oblique line on the thyroid cartilage to the fifth tracheal ring.

III. The thyroid is enclosed within the **pretracheal fascia**. This also encloses the larynx, trachea, pharynx, oesophagus and infrahyoid strap muscles.

IV. The thyroid gland is related posteromedially to the following structures:
- larynx and trachea
- pharynx and oesophagus (note the lateral lobes extend around the trachea to come into contact with the oesophagus)
- recurrent laryngeal nerves.

The carotid sheath is a posterolateral relation.

V. The thyroid gland is supplied by two paired arteries and an inconstant unpaired artery. Each has to be ligated during a total thyroidectomy. More specifically:
- **Superior thyroid artery** (paired) – normally arises as the first branch of the external carotid artery. It descends to pierce the thyroid fascia before dividing into anterior and posterior branches. The anterior branch supplies the anterior surface of the gland, and the posterior branch the lateral and medial surfaces.
- **Inferior thyroid artery** (paired) – this artery arises from the thyrocervical trunk (a branch of the first part of the subclavian artery). It divides outside the pretracheal fascia into multiple branches which supply the inferior and posterior surfaces of the gland, including the parathyroid glands.
- **Thyroid ima artery** (unpaired) – this inconstant branch is present in less than 10% of individuals and arises from either the aortic arch or the brachiocephalic trunk. When present, one or more superior or inferior thyroid arteries may be absent.

VI. Three pairs of veins drain the thyroid gland and each must be ligated in a total thyroidectomy. They are the following:
- The **superior thyroid veins** – these arise from the upper pole of the gland and run with the superior thyroid arteries, draining into the internal jugular veins.
- The **middle thyroid veins** – arise from the lateral surfaces of the gland and also drain into the internal jugular veins.
- The **inferior thyroid veins** – these are formed from a venous plexus below the thyroid gland anterior to the trachea. The inferior thyroid veins drain into their corresponding brachiocephalic veins. Commonly, there is only one inferior thyroid vein, which then drains into the left brachiocephalic vein.

VII. Two nerves lie in close proximity to each lobe of the thyroid gland. Both are at risk of injury during a thyroidectomy. They are the following:
- The **recurrent laryngeal nerve** – the courses of the left and right nerves differ, although both are branches of the corresponding vagus nerve (CN X). The left originates in the thorax and loops under the arch of the aorta, whereas the right originates in the neck and loops under the right subclavian artery. They both ascend in the neck in the tracheo-oesophageal groove and become intimately related to the inferior thyroid arteries.

- The **external branch of the superior laryngeal nerve** – each runs with the superior thyroid artery above the superior pole of the thyroid gland, before turning medially to supply the cricothyroid muscle. The exact position of each varies; however there is an area 1–2 cm from the thyroid capsule where the nerve and vessel are most intimately related.

VIII. To minimise the risk of injury to these nerves during a thyroidectomy, the surgeon must be mindful of the close association of the external branch of the superior laryngeal nerve with the superior thyroid artery, and the recurrent laryngeal nerve with the inferior thyroid artery. Surgical practices differ, but it is often recommended that the superior thyroid artery be ligated close to the thyroid capsule, and the inferior thyroid artery either ligated well laterally or its individual branches ligated on the surface of the thyroid (the latter also maximises preservation of the blood supply to the parathyroids), to reduce the risk of iatrogenic nerve injury.

IX. The **recurrent laryngeal nerve** supplies all the intrinsic muscles of the larynx other than the cricothyroid muscle. If there is a complete palsy of the nerve, the corresponding vocal cord tends to adopt a semi-abducted position; the patient may be asymptomatic or complain of hoarseness. Bilateral palsies may cause stridor with upper airway obstruction.

The **external branch of the superior laryngeal nerve** supplies the cricothyroid muscle which elongates the vocal cords. Inability to lengthen the cords results in a reduced capacity to create high-pitch sounds. The patient may be asymptomatic, especially in unilateral lesions.

X. The thyroid gland is made up of two main types of cells – follicular and parafollicular. The microstructure of the thyroid gland is organised into follicles concerned with the absorption and storage of iodine. The follicles are lined by **follicular cells** which are responsible for producing thyroglobulin (the stored form of triiodothyronine (T_3) and thyroxine (T_4)). Scattered amongst the follicular cells are **parafollicular cells** (C cells) which secrete calcitonin.

XI. There are three main types of cancer that arise from thyroid tissue:

- **papillary carcinoma** (≈80%) – arising from follicular cells and tending to spread via lymphatics;
- **follicular carcinoma** (10–15%) – arising from follicular cells and tending to vascular metastases;
- **medullary** (≈10%) – arising from parafollicular cells and may be associated with multiple endocrine neoplasia type 2 (MEN-2). Can spread by vascular and lymphatic pathways.

Anaplastic carcinomas and other thyroid tumours are rare.

XII. The **parathyroid glands** normally lie on the posterior surface of the gland and each has the appearance of a tan coloured lentil. There are usually two superior and two inferior glands, all supplied by the inferior thyroid artery. Their position is variable, although the superior pair is more constantly sited at the mid-posterior border of the thyroid gland. They secrete parathyroid hormone which is involved in calcium homeostasis.

XIII. See Image 8.3.

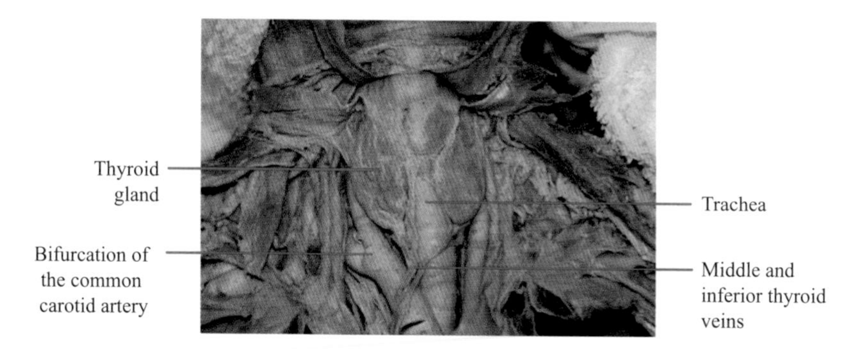

Image 8.3

Question 3

I. The **parotid gland**, the largest of the salivary glands, is an irregular, lobulated, yellowish gland which lies below the external ear anterior to the sternocleidomastoid (SCM), overlapping the ramus of the mandible. The surface markings are as follows:
   - superior – lower border of the zygomatic arch;
   - posterior – external auditory meatus, mastoid process, anterior border of SCM;
   - inferior – a line drawn from the mastoid process to the junction of the body and greater cornu of the hyoid bone;
   - anterior – the gland overlaps the posterior surface of the masseter muscle.

II. The parotid duct, or Stensen's duct,[1] runs from the anterior portion of the parotid gland and opens opposite the second upper molar tooth. The duct lies along the middle third of a line joining the lower border of the tragus (external ear) and the angle of the mouth (commissure). The duct can be palpated as a tubular structure overlying a contracted masseter.

III. Running through the parotid gland are the following structures, arranged from superficial to deep:
   - the **facial nerve** (CN VII);
   - the **retromandibular vein** – formed in the parotid gland by the union of the maxillary and superficial temporal veins;
   - the **external carotid artery** – divides into the maxillary and superficial temporal arteries.

   The auriculotemporal nerve, a branch of the mandibular division of the trigeminal nerve, lies deep to the parotid rather than passing through it. It supplies the gland with postganglionic parasympathetic fibres from the otic ganglion.

IV. Structure A is the **facial nerve**. Once within the parotid gland, the nerve splits into upper and lower trunks and then into its five terminal branches. The five branches leave the gland along its anteromedial surface to innervate the muscles of facial expression.

V. Structure B is the **temporal branch** of the facial nerve. It supplies the auricular muscles, the frontal part of occipitofrontalis, and orbicularis oculi.

VI. The **zygomatic branch** crosses the zygomatic bone and is the dominant supply to orbicularis oculi, which is responsible for closing the eyes.

VII. The **buccal branch** runs alongside the parotid duct. It has superficial and deep branches supplying muscles around the nose and mouth, including buccinator.

VIII. The **marginal mandibular branch** supplies the muscles of the lower lip and chin. It has an important surgical relationship to the lower border of the mandible (see part XIV).

IX. The **cervical branch** supplies platysma and communicates with the transverse cervical nerve.

X. Structure G is the **superficial temporal artery**. A temporal artery biopsy may be performed to confirm a diagnosis of giant cell arteritis.

XI. A lump or swelling of the parotid gland may be classified as **neoplastic** or **non-neoplastic**:

- **Non-neoplastic** lesions include sialadenitis (inflammation), sialolithiasis (stone formation) and swelling due to infection, systemic disease or drug reactions.
- **Neoplastic** lesions can be further sub-classified into benign (the commonest) or malignant. Pain and involvement of the facial nerve suggests a malignant tumour, such as a mucoepidermoid carcinoma, adenoid cystic carcinoma or squamous cell carcinoma. Benign tumours such as pleomorphic adenomas and Warthin's tumours[2] rarely cause pain or involve the facial nerve.

XII. The submandibular gland has two lobes – **superficial** and **deep** – which are demarcated by the posterior border of the **mylohyoid** muscle. The **superficial** lobe lies below and lateral to the mylohyoid, occupies most of the submandibular triangle, and overlaps the edge of the anterior belly of the digastric muscle. The **deep** lobe lies between the mylohyoid and hyoglossus muscles. Posteriorly, the submandibular gland is separated from the parotid gland by the stylomandibular ligament.

XIII. The submandibular duct (also known as Wharton's duct[3]) is approximately 5 cm long and passes forward from the submandibular gland between mylohyoid and hyoglossus to drain into the oral cavity **either side of the frenulum of the tongue**.

XIV. The nerve most at risk is the **marginal mandibular branch** of the facial nerve. It travels anteriorly parallel to the body of the mandible, often running below its lower border (but within 3 cm of it), superficial to the submandibular gland. Incisions approaching the submandibular gland are traditionally placed two fingerbreadths below the body of the mandible to avoid injuring the nerve.

XV. Injury to the marginal mandibular branch of the facial nerve results in the inability to depress the corner of the mouth, which is particularly evident when smiling.

Question 4

I. Structure A is the **common carotid artery**.

II. The common carotid artery bifurcates at the level of the **upper border of the thyroid cartilage**, which equates to the **C3/4 junction**. It can be compressed by pressing it against the prominent anterior tubercle of C6 (at the level of the cricoid cartilage).

III. Structure B is the **external carotid artery**. This can be distinguished from the internal carotid artery, intraoperatively and radiologically, by the presence of branches. The internal carotid artery has no branches in the neck, whereas the external has eight named branches in the head and neck.

IV. The external carotid artery ends by dividing into the **maxillary** and **superficial temporal** arteries. Its other branches, in relation to their origin from the external carotid artery, are:
- anterior – superior thyroid, lingual and facial arteries;
- posterior – occipital and posterior auricular arteries;
- medial – ascending pharyngeal artery.

V. Structure C is the **internal carotid artery**. It has no branches in the neck. Notice it has a stenosis just distal to the bifurcation of the common carotid artery. This could account for the patient's TIA.

VI. The **superior thyroid artery** is usually the first branch of the external carotid artery, arising from its anterior surface. As its name suggests, it supplies the thyroid gland, and also some overlying skin.

VII. D is the **carotid sinus**. This is a small dilation of the origin of the internal carotid artery; **baroreceptors** are present in the wall of the artery at this site. These are supplied by the carotid sinus branch of the glossopharyngeal nerve (CN IX) and the vagus nerve (CN X). Note the difference with the carotid body, which is a small cluster of chemoreceptors located posterior to the carotid bifurcation; this is also supplied by the carotid sinus and vagus nerves.

VIII. The baroreceptors of the carotid sinus have an important role to play in **maintaining arterial blood pressure**. They detect changes in the stretch of the arterial wall and, through neural feedback to the medulla, are able to induce autonomic changes to regulate blood pressure. The other main group of baroreceptors are located in the aortic arch. The chemoreceptors of the carotid body regulate respiration by sensing changes in arterial pH, pCO_2 and pO_2.

IX. The common and internal carotid arteries are enclosed within the **carotid sheath**, a condensation of deep cervical fascia. The sheath is thicker around the arteries than the internal jugular vein, allowing the vein to expand.

X. The contents of the carotid sheath are:
- common and internal **carotid arteries** (medial)
- **internal jugular vein** (lateral)
- **vagus nerve** (between and posterior to the vessels)
- **ansa cervicalis** (superficial to the internal jugular vein).

XI. The right common carotid artery is a branch of the **brachiocephalic trunk**, and the left originates directly from the **arch of the aorta**. The right artery therefore only has a cervical course whereas the left has a thoracic and a cervical course.

XII. The following nerves are particularly at risk of injury during a carotid endarterectomy:
- **Hypoglossal nerve** – this nerve crosses the internal and external carotid arteries above the common carotid bifurcation running forward over the loop of the lingual artery.
- **Vagus nerve** – the vagus nerve runs posterior to the internal/common carotid arteries and the internal jugular vein, within the carotid sheath. Injury to the vagus nerve would mostly manifest through effects on the recurrent laryngeal nerve.
- **Marginal mandibular branch of the facial nerve** – when this nerve runs well below the lower border of the mandible, it is at risk during endarterectomy. For consequences of injury, see Question 3, part XV, in this chapter.
- **Ansa cervicalis** – formed by a superior root (C1) from the hypoglossal nerve and an inferior root (C2,3) from the cervical plexus. The ansa cervicalis is embedded in the anterior wall of the carotid sheath, but injury rarely causes clinical effects.

XIII. Structure A is the cut **lateral end of the clavicle**.

XIV. This is **scalenus medius**, which arises from the transverse processes of the cervical vertebrae and is inserted into the upper surface of the first rib.

XV. Structure C is **scalenus anterior**, which arises from the transverse processes of C3–6 vertebrae and inserts into the scalene tubercle on the inner border of the first rib. It is an important landmark in the root of the neck.

XVI. All the scalene muscles (anterior, middle and posterior) are innervated by the anterior rami of the lower cervical nerves. Scalenus anterior receives branches from **C4–6**.

XVII. The roots of the brachial plexus emerge between the anterior and middle scalene muscles. Label D points to the **trunks of the brachial plexus**; these run in the posterior triangle of the neck.

XVIII. This is the **subclavian artery**, which also passes between the anterior and middle scalene muscles. The right subclavian artery is a branch of the brachiocephalic trunk, whereas the left is a direct branch off the arch of the aorta. At the outer border of the first rib, the subclavian artery becomes the axillary artery.

XIX. The thoracic outlet, or superior thoracic aperture, is the opening through which the neck communicates with the thorax. Its boundaries are:

Table 8.2

Type	Structure involved	Pathology
Neogenic (>80%)	Brachial plexus	Aberrant or hypertrophied scalene muscles, classically in swimmers, or cervical ribs/fibrous bands. Compresses the brachial plexus, especially the lower trunk
Venous	Subclavian vein	Usually caused by compression between the costoclavicular ligament and the subclavius muscle
Arterial	Subclavian artery	Usually caused by compression of the second part of the artery by a cervical rib or an abnormal first rib

- posterior – the first thoracic vertebra (T1)
- lateral – the first pair of ribs and their costal cartilages
- anterior – superior border of the manubrium.

XX. Thoracic outlet obstruction syndrome results from compression of neurovascular structures at the thoracic outlet or just beyond. Three distinct clinical pictures exist based on the dominant structures involved. They are described in Table 8.2.

Question 5

I. Structure 1 is the **vocal cord** or **fold.**

II. The **posterior cricoarytenoid muscles** are the only muscles that are able to abduct the vocal cords.

Table 8.3

Muscle	Innervation	Action
Cricothyroid	External laryngeal nerve	Lengthens and stretches the vocal cords
Lateral cricoarytenoid	Recurrent laryngeal nerve	Adducts and shortens the vocal cords, closing the rima glottidis (the opening between the vocal folds and the arytenoid cartilages)
Oblique arytenoid and aryepiglottic	Recurrent laryngeal nerve	Adduct the aryepiglottic folds, acting as a sphincter to the laryngeal inlet
Transverse arytenoid	Recurrent laryngeal nerve	Draws the arytenoid cartilages towards each other, narrowing the rima glottidis
Thyroarytenoid and vocalis	Recurrent laryngeal nerve	Change the pitch and timbre of the voice by drawing the arytenoid cartilages towards the thyroid cartilage, approximating and shortening the vocal cords

The other intrinsic laryngeal muscles are given in Table 8.3.

III. The posterior cricoarytenoid muscles are supplied by the **recurrent laryngeal nerve.**
IV. Structure 2 is the **vestibular fold** (false vocal cord).
V. Structure 3 is the **epiglottis,** which is composed of elastic fibrocartilage.
VI. During deglutition (swallowing), the larynx is elevated and the epiglottis folds back over the glottis. This allows liquids and solids to slide over its smooth mucous membrane, steering them away from entering the larynx.
VII. This is the **aryepiglottic fold,** containing muscular and ligamentous fibres. It covers the upper border of the quadrangular membrane.
VIII. Structure 5 is the mucosa overlying the **arytenoid cartilage,** a pyramidal cartilage sitting on the upper border of the cricoid lamina. The cuneiform and corniculate cartilages lie superiorly.
IX. This is the **piriform fossa** lying on either side of the laryngeal inlet. Ingested liquids and solids are deflected laterally by the epiglottis into the piriform fossae.
X. The **internal laryngeal nerve** lies deep to the mucous membrane of the piriform fossa. This supplies laryngeal sensation above the vocal cords.
XI. Structure 7 is the dorsum of the tongue.

Question 6

I. A is the **foramen lacerum.** This is closed over by fibrous tissue and only transmits a small emissary vein. The internal carotid artery enters the skull through the carotid canal before turning anteromedially above the foramen lacerum to traverse the cavernous sinus.
II. B is the **foramen ovale** which transmits the following structures:
   - mandibular division of the trigeminal nerve
   - lesser petrosal nerve
   - an accessory meningeal branch of the maxillary artery.
III. C is the **foramen spinosum** through which the middle meningeal artery passes.
IV. D is the exit of the **carotid canal** from the petrous temporal bone. It transmits the internal carotid artery and sympathetic nerves.
V. E is the **jugular foramen.** Several important structures pass through this foramen in separate dural compartments. They include:
   - inferior petrosal sinus and glossopharyngeal nerve (anterior compartment);
   - vagus and accessory nerves (middle compartment);
   - sigmoid sinus/internal jugular vein (posterior compartment).
VI. F is the **hypoglossal canal.** This foramen transmits the:
   - hypoglossal nerve (CN XII)
   - meningeal branch of the ascending pharyngeal artery.

VII. The **hypoglossal nerve** (CN XII) is purely motor, although it is accompanied by sensory nerves from the C2 spinal nerve. It supplies all the intrinsic and extrinsic muscles of the tongue, except for palatoglossus (supplied by the vagus nerve).

VIII. G is the **foramen magnum**, which transmits the following structures:
- medulla oblongata (lower end)
- vertebral arteries
- anterior and posterior spinal arteries
- spinal roots of the accessory nerves (CN XI).

IX. 1 is the **frontal bone**, an unpaired bone making up the forehead and most of the anterior cranial fossa.

X. 2 is the **sphenoid bone**, a butterfly-shaped bone consisting of a central body (which contains the pituitary gland) and two lateral wing-like extensions (greater and lesser) on each side. In the illustration, the greater wing of the sphenoid bone is being identified.

XI. 3 is the **temporal bone**. This is a complex bone made up of four parts: squamous temporal, tympanic, petromastoid and styloid process.

XII. 4 is the **occipital bone**, a large bone which contributes to the formation of the posterior cranial fossa and surrounds the foramen magnum.

XIII. The trigeminal nerve has both sensory and motor fibres, but the latter are distributed only with the mandibular division. The three components of CN V are as follows:

a. **Ophthalmic nerve** – this is a purely sensory nerve which passes through the superior orbital fissure to supply the skin over the forehead, scalp, upper eyelids and most of the external nose. It also supplies the eyeball, upper conjunctiva, lacrimal glands, nasal mucosa and frontal sinus.

b. **Maxillary nerve** – this is also a sensory nerve and passes through the foramen rotundum in the floor of the middle cranial fossa. It supplies the skin over the upper lip, lower eyelid and conjunctiva, cheek, maxillary sinus, upper dentition, and parts of the nose and temple.

c. **Mandibular nerve** – this passes through the foramen ovale where it is joined by the small motor root. The sensory component innervates the skin over the mandible (excluding the angle which is supplied by the great auricular nerve, C2,3), lower dentition, floor of the mouth and tongue, and parts of the auricle and temple. The motor component supplies the muscles of mastication, i.e. masseter, temporalis and pterygoid (medial and lateral) muscles, together with the mylohyoid and anterior belly of digastric.

To examine the function of the trigeminal nerve you must test the sensation in all three sensory areas of the nerve (including the cornea) and also check for motor function by assessing masseter and temporalis.

XIV. H is the **frontal bone**.

XV. I is the **nasal septum** (the perpendicular plate of the ethmoid is indicated).
XVI. J is the **zygomatic bone**.
XVII. K is the **maxilla**.
XVIII. L is the **mandible**.
XIX. M indicates the **infraorbital foramen**, which transmits the **infraorbital vessels** and **infraorbital nerve** (the continuation of the maxillary nerve).
XX. The **facial artery**, a branch of the external carotid artery, ascends in this region, having crossed the lower border of the mandible where its pulsation can be felt at the anterior border of masseter. It has a tortuous course towards the medial angle of the eye and supplies much of the skin and muscles of the face.
XXI. O is the **mental foramen** which transmits the **mental nerve** and **vessels**. The mental nerve is a branch of the inferior alveolar nerve (a branch of the mandibular division of the trigeminal nerve) and supplies sensation to the skin of the chin and mucous membrane of the lower lip and gum.

ENDNOTES

1 Niels Stensen (1638–1686), Danish anatomist and Saint.
2 Aldred Scott Warthin (1866–1931), American pathologist.
3 Thomas Wharton (1614–1673), English physician and anatomist.

Index